50 of the Best Snowshoe Trails around Lake Tahoe

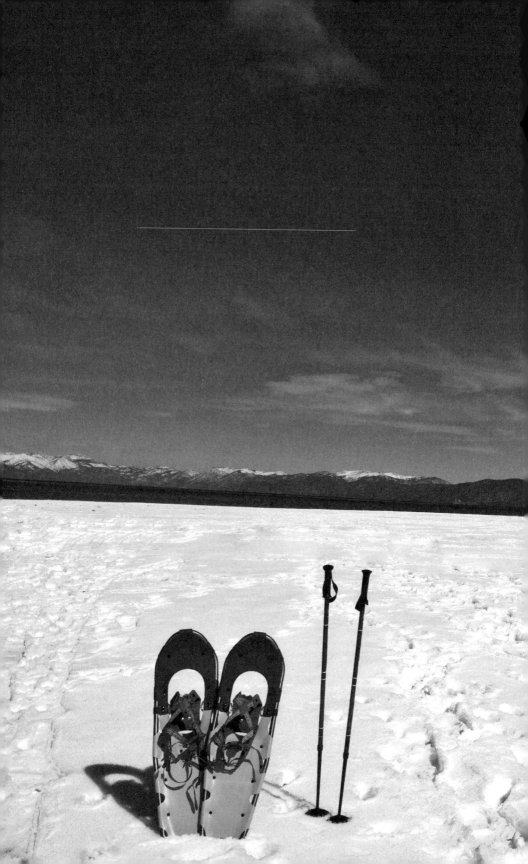

50 of the Best Snowshoe Trails around Lake Tahoe

MIKE WHITE

UNIVERSITY OF NEVADA PRESS *Reno & Las Vegas*

University of Nevada Press | Reno, Nevada 89557 USA
www.unpress.nevada.edu
Copyright © 2018 by University of Nevada Press
All rights reserved
All photographs courtesy of Mike White unless otherwise noted
Adobe Stock: p xi © Oleksandr Dibrova; p 30 © lolo2013

Library of Congress Cataloging-in-Publication Data
Names: White, Michael C., 1952– author.
Title: 50 of the best snowshoe trails around Lake Tahoe / by Mike White.
Other titles: Fifty of the best snowshoe trails around Lake Tahoe
Description: First Edition. | Reno, Nevada : University of Nevada Press, [2018] | Includes index. |
Identifiers: LCCN 2018003958 (print) | LCCN 2018007092 (e-book) |
    ISBN 978-1-943859-79-5 (paper : alk. paper) | ISBN 978-1-943859-80-1 (e-book)
Subjects: LCSH: Snowshoes and snowshoeing—Tahoe, Lake, Region (Calif. and Nev.)—
    Guidebooks. | Cross-country ski trails—Tahoe, Lake, Region (Calif. and Nev.)—
    Guidebooks. | Tahoe, Lake, Region (Calif. and Nev.)—Guidebooks.
Classification: LCC GV853 (e-book) | LCC GV853 .W53 2018 (print) |
    DDC 796.9/20979438—dc23
LC record available at https://lccn.loc.gov/2018003958

The paper used in this book meets the requirements of American National Standard
for Information Sciences—Permanence of Paper for Printed Library Materials,
ANSI/NISO z39.48-1992 (R2002).

Second Printing

Manufactured in the United States of America

Contents

PART FOUR — WEST TAHOE

Illustrations

Photos

Thanks to the love and support of my wife, Robin,
without whom none of my projects would ever make it to print.
I very much appreciated company on the trail from
Keith Catlin, Dal and Candy Hunter, and Bruce Farenkopf.
Many thanks also to the staff at University of Nevada Press
for their efforts.

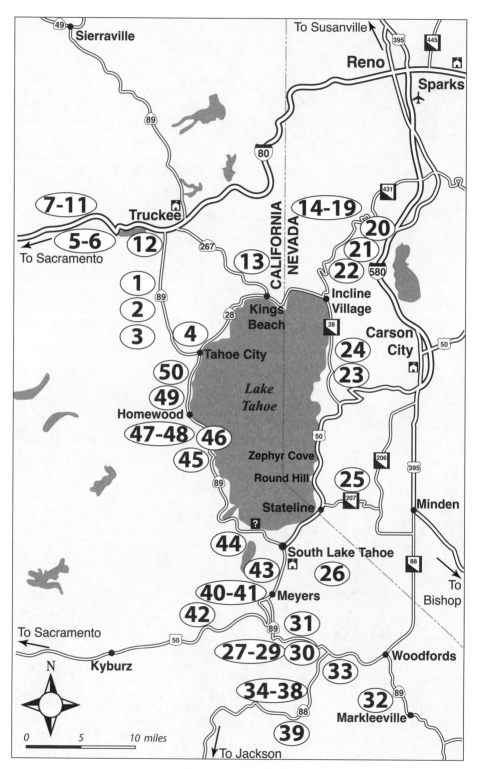

Tahoe Snowshoe Trails

Introduction

Known for the crystal clarity of its deep-blue waters, Lake Tahoe is one of the most spectacular gems in the treasury of the Sierra Nevada. While jewelers measure precious stones in carats, less romantic units of measurement attempt to capture the magnitude of Tahoe's greatness: Twenty-one miles long and twelve miles wide, Tahoe is the largest natural freshwater subalpine lake by volume in North America (outside of Alaska) and, at a depth of 1,645 feet, it is the fourth deepest in North America. Circling the shoreline requires a 72-mile journey. While numbers quantify its size, they seem wholly inadequate at expressing the sublime beauty of the lake and the surrounding landscape.

This large body of water was originally called Lake Bonpland by the famous western explorer, John C. Fremont, for noted French botanist Aimé Jacques Alexandre Bonpland. After first appearing on a map of the area in 1848, the name lasted less than a decade, replaced by Lake Bigler in 1857. A former governor of California, "Bigler" lasted a relatively short time as well, fading away as his reputation became increasingly sullied. By the early 1860s a groundswell had begun for changing the name to the current appellation, "Tahoe," a less then perfect English adaptation of the Washoe word for "big water." Although imperfect, the sentiment seems to capture some of the essence of the huge lake.

As the usually pleasant days of early autumn fade into fall and in turn the autumn leaves littering the ground herald the approach of winter, the attention of outdoor enthusiasts turns toward snowy pursuits. With white powder eventually blanketing the landscape, vehicle access to Tahoe's backcountry becomes more limited and the mountainous terrain around the lake opens up a whole new world of recreational possibilities, particularly for those willing to travel under their own power. Deep-cut canyons, frozen subalpine lakes, knife-edged peaks, and incomparable views are all present in abundance, waiting to be discovered by snowshoers, cross-country and backcountry skiers, and snowboarders. Seemingly never too far out of sight, the cobalt-blue, sparkling waters of Lake Tahoe act as nature's grand mirror, reflecting the glistening, snow-covered terrain circling its basin. Such spectacular scenery combines with the traditionally fair Sierra weather to create a dazzling paradise for winter enthusiasts. Those who visit the area for the first time are often awestruck by the unparalleled beauty around them.

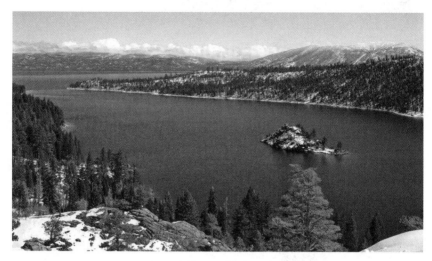

Emerald Bay and Lake Tahoe

Recreation is an important part of life at Lake Tahoe, deemed as Northern California's premier winter playground. More than a dozen alpine ski resorts are scattered around the lake, combined with several cross-country ski centers, and a number of snowmobile concessions. A weekend of pleasant weather will see many families from the Bay Area, Sacramento Valley, western Nevada, and from all around the world engaged in winter pursuits, sledding down hillsides, building snowmen, or gleefully engaged in snowball fights. Seemingly everyone enjoys winters at Lake Tahoe.

Not everything at Lake Tahoe is about frivolity, though, as the sensitive environment in the basin has received much attention in recent decades. Under the banner of "Keep Tahoe Blue," bumper stickers, license plates, and advertisements alert residents and visitors alike to the potential threats to the quality of life here at the lake. Concerns about water quality, air pollution, forest health, and congestion have resulted in some restrictions, and there will most likely be more in the future. Currently, most winter recreationists are free from most of these restrictions, aside from purchasing a SNO-PARK pass, or obtaining a wilderness permit for entry into Desolation Wilderness. However, all outdoor users should observe minimum-impact practices and treat the area with the utmost care when recreating in the Tahoe area. Lake Tahoe and the surrounding region is a tremendous resource, deserving appreciation and respect by all who live, work, and play there.

■ Access

A reasonably adequate network of state and federal highways surrounds Lake Tahoe—although Bay Area residents crawling down Interstate 80 toward home on Sunday night after a weekend of skiing might beg to differ. Weather permitting, these roads remain open throughout the winter, closing only during the most severe winter storms. The lone exception is the stretch of state highway around Emerald Bay, where avalanches may close the road for significant periods after major snowfalls.

Interstate 80 provides the principal gateway to the Tahoe area from Northern California. The four-lane highway gradually ascends the west slope beyond the Sacramento Valley and reaches the Sierra crest at 7,227-foot Donner Summit, before plummeting more steeply along the Truckee River to Reno-Sparks. Replaced by I-80 in the early 1960s, the two-lane Lincoln Highway (Old State Route 40) was an engineering marvel at the time of construction. The old road mostly parallels the modern interstate and continues to provide unhurried motorists with exceptional roadside scenery.

U.S. Highway 50, the first paved transcontinental road in America, provides the principal access to Tahoe at the south end of the lake. The mostly two-lane road bears travelers east from the Sacramento Valley and over 7,377-foot Echo Summit on the way to Lake Tahoe. From the south shore, a four-lane stretch of highway follows the lakeshore through the casino district and around the southeast side of the lake before ascending to 7,146-foot Spooner Summit and then descending to Carson City and a junction with Interstate 580. Of the three major east-west thoroughfares affording access to the Tahoe area, Highway 50 is the only one that actually reaches the shore.

Leaving the Sacramento Valley near the town of Jackson, State Route 88 follows a sometimes-winding route on the way to 8,593-foot Carson Pass, about 15 air miles from the south shore of Lake Tahoe. The highest of the three major east-west highways, the altitude combined with some favorable topography creates a winter wonderland for recreationists around the pass. Continuing east, the two-lane highway drops in dramatic fashion toward Carson Valley and the neighboring Nevada towns of Minden and Gardnerville.

A continuous band of pavement follows a rough oval around the entire shoreline of Lake Tahoe. Although composed of segments of four separate highways (CA 89, U.S. 50, NV 28, and CA 28), in practicality, the route forms an uninterrupted loop all the way around the lake. Various secondary highways, along with previously mentioned Highway 50, make connections from points beyond Tahoe to this loop. From Truckee, two state highways leave Interstate 80 and connect to the loop at the north end of the lake. From the west side of Truckee, California State Route 89 follows the Truckee River upstream past turnoffs to Squaw Valley and Alpine Meadows to the river's gates at Tahoe City. From the east side of Truckee, California State Route 267 passes through Martis Valley, climbs to 7,179-foot Brockway Summit, and then descends to the lakeshore at Kings Beach. From the south side of Reno, Nevada's State Route 431 (Mount Rose Highway) heads southwest from I-580 and follows a winding climb past Mount Rose Ski Tahoe to 8,933-foot Mount Rose Summit, making this road the highest winter-maintained crossing of the Sierra Nevada Range. From there, the highway drops past Tahoe Meadows and continues to Incline Village and a junction with Nevada State Route 28. Known locally as Kingsbury Grade, State Route 207 climbs steeply from the west side of Carson Valley to 7,344-foot Daggett Pass and then descends to a connection with U.S. 50 at Stateline. From Meyers, California State Route 89 leaves U.S. 50 and climbs southbound to 7,735-foot Luther Pass before dropping shortly to a junction with California State Route 88 in Hope Valley.

Transportation
Automobiles
As with many recreation areas of the West, access to ski and snowshoe trails described in this guide is primarily via private automobile. Rental car companies service Reno-Tahoe International Airport, South Lake Tahoe Airport, and Truckee Tahoe Airport, as well as cities and towns nearby. Although mass transit options have improved over the years at Lake Tahoe, getting to trailheads without driving a vehicle is no easy task for the majority of routes described in this guide.

Local Bus Service
NORTH SHORE: TART (Tahoe Area Regional Transit) offers bus service for the northwest shore of the lake on three routes. The Mainline Route connects Incline Village to Tahoma. The California State Route 267 route runs between Crystal Bay and Truckee (Amtrak station), accessing Northstar and the Truckee Tahoe Airport on the way. The California State Route 89 route runs between Truckee (Amtrak station) and Tahoe City, accessing Squaw Valley on the way. On weekends and holiday weeks between late December and early April, TART offers a free skiers' shuttle with stops between Incline Village and Tahoe City to Squaw Valley, Alpine Meadows, and Homewood ski areas. For more information visit www.placer.ca.gov.

SOUTH SHORE: The Tahoe Transportation District offers bus service in the South Lake Tahoe and Stateline areas on **BlueGO**. A ski shuttle operates during the winter to the California and Nevada sides of Heavenly Lake Tahoe ski resort. For more information visit http://www.tahoetransportation.org /transit/south-shore-services.

Ski Shuttle Buses

RENO: A variety of shuttle bus services extend to most of Tahoe's downhill resorts from both major casino/hotels in Reno and Lake Tahoe. Reservations are strongly recommended.

Mount Rose Ski Tahoe operates a shuttle between Reno hotels and the resort on Saturdays and holiday weekends (www.skirose.com/plan-your-trip /shuttles).

North Lake Tahoe Express has three routes connecting the Reno-Tahoe International Airport to a variety of north shore destinations, including Squaw Valley and Northstar ski resorts, Truckee Tahoe Airport, and the Truckee Amtrak station (www.northlaketahoeexpress.com).

Patty's Tours connects Reno-Tahoe International Airport and major casino/hotels directly to Northstar and Squaw Valley ski resorts. Round-trip only. Visit www.pattystours.com/skishuttle.html.

South Tahoe Airporter runs between Reno-Tahoe International Airport and major hotels in South Lake Tahoe (www.southtahoeexpress.com).

TAHOE: Almost all of the Tahoe area ski resorts offer some type of shuttle service from major Lake Tahoe communities, some of which are free. In addition, shuttles can also be reserved from Bay Area and Sacramento locations. Consult the individual resort websites for more information.

Bus Lines

Greyhound offers service to Truckee and Reno. Visit www.greyhound.com for more information.

Railroads

Amtrak's California Zephyr makes daily stops in Reno, Truckee, Colfax, Roseville, Sacramento, Davis, Martinez, Richmond, and Emeryville. Visit www .amtrak.com for more information.

Major Airports

San Francisco, Oakland, and Sacramento all have international airports, but the closest major airport to the Lake Tahoe region is Reno-Tahoe International Airport.

Municipal Airports

Carson City, Douglas County (Gardnerville), Truckee Tahoe, and South Lake Tahoe are light-duty airports, primarily serving private aircraft or charter service.

■ Lodging and Dining

A plethora of lodging and dining options are available in and around the Lake Tahoe area, although you should expect to pay premium prices during the busy ski season.

Campgrounds

Winter closes most of the government and private campgrounds that serve the hordes of summer visitors around Lake Tahoe. A few do remain open year-round for the hardy campers who don't faint at the idea of camping in cold temperatures.

Davis Creek Regional Park: Located on Nevada State Route 429, just west of I-580 in Washoe Valley, about 16 miles south of Reno (www.washoecounty parks.com).

Ed Z'berg Sugar Pine Point State Park: Located on the west shore, 2.5 miles south of Homewood (www.parks.ca.gov).

Grover Hot Springs State Park: About 9 miles west of Markleeville (www.parks.ca.gov).

Lakeside Mobile Home & RV Park: Located in South Lake Tahoe, 3 miles west of Stateline on Cedar Avenue (530-544-4704).

Washoe Lake State Park: Located on Nevada State Route 428 east of I-580 about 7 miles north of Carson City (www.parks.nv.gov).

Zephyr Cove RV Park & Campgrounds: Located on the east shore, 4 miles north of Stateline (www.zephyrcove.com).

■ Winter Travel

Having lived at the eastern base of the Sierra since the mid-1970s, a half hour's drive from Tahoe's north shore, I have experienced a number of winters, concluding that "normal" is a statistical average rarely coinciding with the weather of the real world. Winter weather has spanned the climatic spectrum from Godzilla El Niños, which produced winter-like conditions all the way to the beginning of summer, to multiyear droughts, when hiking the Tahoe Rim Trail on bare ground was possible in January.

■ Weather

Despite the scientific advances in long-range forecasting, determining what the winter will bring to the Lake Tahoe region is somewhat difficult until the season actually unfolds. Fortunately, these days reliable short-term forecasts are readily available to virtually anyone with access to a computer, smart phone, or television. Especially during the winter, recreationists venturing into the backcountry should do so only when armed with a reliable and current forecast.

Wild variations aside, the climate of Lake Tahoe can be classified on the whole as dry. The sun shines 84 percent of the time, an average of 307 days per year. Many an ideal trip occurs during days of bright sunshine following a storm blanketing the Sierra with a layer of fresh powder.

Typically, winter storms bringing moisture to the Tahoe basin plow into the Sierra Nevada from the west, dropping snow on the higher elevations before moving east across the Great Basin. Most of these storms last no more than a day or two, separated by stable periods of dry, mostly sunny weather. However, severe storms lasting for days that dump incredible amounts of snow are quite possible (1997–1998, 2004–2005, 2010–2011, and 2016–2017, for recent examples). Some winter days the weather at Lake Tahoe is idyllic, other times life-threatening. Remember, this is where the epic struggle of the Donner Party took place.

Average seasonal snowfall measures nearly 190 inches at lake level and substantially greater at higher elevations (ski resorts have reported as much as 300 to 500 inches per season—over 600 inches in some locations during the record-setting winter of 2016–2017). Typically, snow occurs between November and April, with the heaviest amounts usually from December through March. However, snowfall has been recorded during every month of the year at one time or another. Winter daytime temperatures at lake level are relatively mild, with average highs around 40 degrees Fahrenheit and average lows around 20 degrees Fahrenheit.

Although firm guarantees are nonexistent, sunshine and mild temperatures are a reasonable expectation for a day of snowshoeing, skiing, or boarding in the Tahoe Sierra. However, all recreationists must be prepared for all conditions—sunshine, snow, sleet, rain, wind, and cold can be extreme at any time. Wild variations in the weather may even occur during the same day, sometimes within hours. Residents commenting on the weather to outsiders will often be heard to say, "If you don't like the weather, wait five minutes." Make sure you have with you the appropriate clothing and equipment to successfully endure whatever conditions you might possibly encounter.

■ SEASON

The winter snowpack may vary greatly from one year to the next, making accurate predictions for when the best conditions exist for snow sports quite difficult. Typically, there is enough snow at lake level for these activities from December through March. During years of abundant early snowfall, the season may begin as early as November and, if the snow continues, extend through April or even into May or June. With such a preponderance of alpine resorts rimming the basin, getting a current snow report is straightforward from their websites.

Snow conditions around the lake will vary due to a variety of factors. Altitude is an important determiner of both the quantity and quality of the snowpack. During warm periods, the snow around the shores of Lake Tahoe (6,200 feet) may be a wet mush, while 2,000 feet higher at Carson Pass conditions might be excellent. Geographical position also plays an important part in snowfall distribution. As Pacific storms approach the Tahoe area from the ocean, rising clouds typically deposit more snow on the Sierra crest than what is left to fall on the Carson Range farther east. Exposure, or aspect to the sun, also affects snow conditions, as south-facing slopes receive the most direct sunlight, followed by west-, east-, and finally north-facing slopes. Forested areas, where branches block the sun from the forest floor, will hang onto the snow longer than open meadows and exposed hillsides. Topography, wind patterns, and microclimates are additional factors influencing snow conditions. All of these components combine to make forecasting the quality and quantity of the snowpack a highly variable speculation.

These factors must be considered when trying to determine the best time to take a trip into the winter backcountry. A wise adventurer consults the avalanche, weather, and ski reports before venturing out into the snowy terrain around Lake Tahoe. Additionally, checking in with staff at Forest Service ranger stations may be helpful.

■ Route Finding

No backcountry skill is more important in winter than the ability to find your way over snow-covered terrain safely to your destination and back. Unlike the summer hiking season, there are no trails to follow, unless opting for the safety of following a marked trail at a resort. Even if you have the luxury of following the tracks of a previous party, those can easily be obscured by a fifteen-minute snowfall. Without the presence of a well-marked route, you must be able to interpret major and minor features of the terrain, accurately read a map, competently use a compass or GPS device, and navigate through the backcountry for most of the trips described in this book. Space does not allow for a thorough dissertation on all the necessary elements of navigation, orienteering, and route finding, so you must gain an understanding of these skills from other sources. The following principles should serve as a general outline of a more detailed comprehension of this art.

- Study the route thoroughly before leaving home.
- Leave a detailed description of the proposed route and a timeline with a reliable person, along with what agency to contact if that becomes necessary.
- Carry a topographic map of the area, compass, and GPS receiver and know how to use them.

- Constantly observe the terrain as you travel and mentally note major and minor features along the way.
- If necessary, mark the trail (removing markers on the return trip).
- Everyone in the party should travel together at all times.

Note: While using electronics, such as GPS receivers, personal locators, cell phones, and so on, may be helpful, no piece of equipment is an adequate replacement for the skills of navigation, orienteering, and routefinding.

Objective Hazards

Sun

For most people, the best days for winter pursuits in the mountains around Lake Tahoe occur on "bluebird days," when the snow is fresh and the skies are crystal clear. Unfortunately, these conditions may produce their own set of problems: sun, snow, and altitude combine to create the perfect reflective oven for baking exposed skin and damaging eyes. While winter finds most recreationists fully covered by some sort of apparel, the face is often the exception. Apply an effective sunblock to all exposed areas of skin and reapply as necessary to avoid sunburn from the intense rays of the sun.

Snow blindness is a very real problem at these elevations on sunny days. This malady is caused by prolonged exposure of the eyes to ultraviolet rays. Wear an effective pair of sunglasses or goggles that filter out at least 90 percent of UVA and UVB rays. Make sure your eye protection adequately covers rays coming in from the side as well.

Dehydration

Becoming dehydrated in the midst of so much frozen water may seem counterintuitive, but without drinking enough water to replenish fluids lost through respiration and perspiration during vigorous winter activities, you may put yourself at risk. Pack and drink plenty of fluids while snowshoeing, skiing, or boarding, as most water sources are frozen and eating snow is an inadequate long-term option. If open water happens to exist, be aware that many water sources in the Tahoe area may be contaminated with pathogens and should be treated before drinking.

Altitude

Most elevations around Lake Tahoe are not considered extreme. However, some people, particularly those living at or near sea level, may suffer the effects of altitude sickness, which can take the form of three syndromes: acute mountain sickness, high-altitude pulmonary edema (HAPE), and high-altitude cerebral edema (HACE). Symptoms of altitude sickness include headache, fatigue, loss of appetite, shortness of breath, nausea, vomiting, drowsiness, dizziness, memory loss, and loss of mental acuity. Although very rare at these elevations, being afflicted with altitude sickness, which can result in death, is a remote possibility if preventative action is not taken.

To avoid these maladies, drink plenty of fluids, eat plenty of carbohydrates, and acclimatize slowly. A rapid descent will usually resolve any of the aforementioned symptoms. A severe case of altitude sickness is unlikely at these elevations during one-day trips, although not impossible.

Cold

Hypothermia is a condition in which the human body's core temperature drops below normal in response to prolonged exposure to cold. This happens when the body loses heat faster than it can produce it. Air temperature is not always the determining factor, as many cases of hypothermia occur when the thermometer registers temperatures above freezing. Wind chill, fatigue, and wetness (from exposure to rain, melting snow, submersion, or even excessive perspiration) may contribute to hypothermia. As body temperature drops, the heart, nervous system, and internal organs fail to work properly. Without proper treatment, heart failure, respiratory failure, and even death can occur.

The best solution for avoiding hypothermia is prevention. Don't become too tired, too wet, or too cold. Dress in layers made of appropriate fabrics and take the time to adjust your clothing to changing conditions, preventing yourself from becoming too cold as well as impeding excessive wetness, from either precipitation or perspiration. Refrain from pushing on toward exhaustion. Drink plenty of fluids and eat plenty of energy-producing food. Carry extra clothes in your vehicle in case you need to change out of wet clothes for the ride home. If you suspect someone in your party is showing signs of hypothermia, handle the situation immediately. Due to loss in mental acuity, you won't be able to detect symptoms in yourself.

Frostbite, a condition in which human tissue actually freezes from prolonged exposure to cold, is a potential concern during winter. The most susceptible areas include feet, hands, faces, and ears. As temperatures are rarely extreme in the generally mild Sierra Nevada, adequate equipment, such as properly fitting winter footwear, warm socks, gloves, and hat should counteract the prolonged exposure to cold that can cause this malady.

Avalanches

Perhaps the most impressive winter hazard in the backcountry is the avalanche. Space does not allow a comprehensive treatise on avalanches, but plenty of resources exist for gaining a better understanding of their causes. Avalanches usually occur due to the instability between the surface layer and the underlying snow, which may exist for a variety of reasons. They most commonly occur during and soon after storms, or during periods of rising temperatures, but are not limited to these conditions.

The most avalanche-prone areas include gullies, moderate-angle slopes between 30 and 45 degrees, north-facing slopes in winter, south-facing slopes in spring, lee slopes, treeless slopes, and hillsides where younger trees are bordered by more mature forest. In addition, hillsides with a convex slope are prone to fracture more easily than ones with a concave slope. As much as is feasible, avoid these areas, particularly during periods of instability.

Many experts have put forth theories about what to do if caught in an avalanche. My own limited experience, along with reports from others, leads me to believe that the majority of avalanches happen far too quickly and with too much force for an unfortunate victim to do much of anything of consequence. However, conventional wisdom dictates that a victim should attempt to get on their back with head uphill and make a swimming motion with their arms in an attempt to stay on top of the snow. Working over toward the edge of the slide is also recommended, if possible. Good luck! Like so many things in life, the best solution is to avoid the problem altogether. The following guidelines will help to minimize avalanche danger.

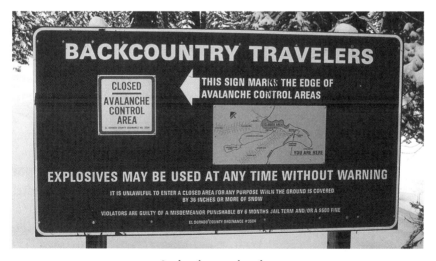

Avalanche warning sign

> **AN UNEXPECTED RIDE BELOW SAWTOOTH RIDGE.** Even small avalanches can pack a considerable wallop. Many years ago after a successful spring climb on Dragtooth on Sawtooth Ridge above Twin Lakes outside of Bridgeport, we decided to glissade down a snow-filled gully as our descent route. After a prolonged period of questioning the wisdom of such an action, I dropped to my rear end and pushed off down the gully. About halfway downslope I felt a push from behind and quickly started to somersault down the gully, coming to rest at the base, stripped of my hat, gloves, and backpack, the apparel and equipment scattered haphazardly across the snow. My outer parka was halfway over my head and snow filled every conceivable passageway through my remaining clothing. After gathering my wits and surveying the situation, I realized that this tremendous force, which had tossed me and my equipment across the mountain like a rag doll, was created by an avalanche a mere 12 inches high and about 6 feet across—an extremely minor avalanche.

- Obtain the current avalanche report (530-587-3558 extension 258, or www.sierraavalanchecenter.org).
- Select the safest route—avoid avalanche-prone areas.
- Test slopes for stability.
- Carry the proper equipment and know how to use it (may include shovels, probes, transceivers, airbag packs, avalanche cord, cell phone, first-aid kit).
- Attend a Level One avalanche course, which not only teaches about avalanches but also how to make good decisions in the winter backcountry.

Cornices

Another potentially impressive feature of the winter landscape is the cornice, an overhanging ledge of snow at the crest of a ridge formed when prevailing winds distribute accumulating snowfall leeward over the edge. Cornices pose two potential problems. Eventually and without warning, cornices may break off and plunge to the slope below, possibly triggering avalanches on unstable slopes. Obviously, the larger the cornice, the greater potential exists for calamity. A less obvious but just as dangerous problem arises when you're traveling along a ridge and venture on top of the overhanging cornice—you may suddenly break through and go for an unexpected and possibly fatal fall.

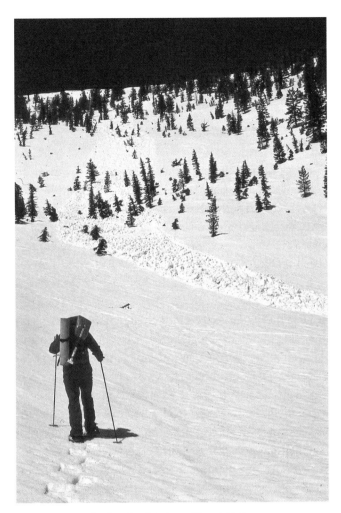
Avalanche debris on Mount Tallac

Trail Etiquette

Generally, trail etiquette is much the same in winter as in summer. Follow minimum-impact techniques just as you would on a summer hike or back-packing trip. Observing the following additional winter guidelines should help you to be a considerate and responsible trail user.

Snowshoers should avoid walking in the tracks of skiers. This allows skiers to reuse their tracks for return trips and preserves the existing track for future skiers.

Snowshoers should yield the right of way to skiers, as snowshoers should have more control over their movements than skiers. Both snowshoers and skiers should yield to snowmobiles in multiuse areas for obvious reasons.

Keep pets and their products under control. Many winter recreationists share their winter backcountry adventures with their dogs. For those who do, ensure your dog is well socialized and is under voice control. Dog owners are also responsible for packing out their pet's solid waste—few things are more unsightly in the winter backcountry than popular areas littered with dog feces.

■ Sanitation

Winter presents a whole different situation for dealing with the proper disposal of human waste materials. Urinating is fairly straightforward—as long as you don't pee into the snow above a lake or stream. Other than protecting water sources, visual appearance is the main consideration. Find a location well off obvious routes, or away from campsites if you're winter camping, to avoid visual pollution. Peeing into a tree well is often a preferred location. When finished urinating, spread some snow over the top to reduce the appearance.

Defecating in the winter backcountry is not nearly as benign as urinating. Short of removing the waste altogether, which remains to most users as an undesirable alternative, there is really no adequate way to dispose of human feces that doesn't adversely affect the environment in some way. Burying stool in the soil at warmer times of the year allows it to gradually decompose and, when a suitable site is used, provides minimal risk of groundwater contamination. The danger of defecating in the snow in winter occurs during the spring, when melting snow transports an excessive amount of the stool into water sources. Some experts have attributed the rise in giardia in the backcountry to the poor sanitation practices of winter users.

So then, what should be done? Taking care of business before or after a visit to the backcountry certainly avoids the problem altogether. However, if nature calls at a less opportune time, the best solution is to pack it out. For those who are not blessed with the ability to regulate their stools and have no desire to pack out their waste, there are a few practical guidelines.

- Pick a site well away from traveled areas and potential campsites.
- Choose a location that won't obviously contaminate a water source.
- Find a southern exposure and position the stool just below the surface (this allows sunlight and the freeze-thaw cycle to begin the decomposition process).
- Pack out used toilet paper in a sealable plastic bag.

Although this guide is primarily concerned with day users, overnighters should use consideration when disposing of wastewater and leftover food.

Permits
Wilderness Permits
Desolation Wilderness: A valid wilderness permit is required year-round in Desolation Wilderness for all day trips and overnight stays. Day users can obtain free permits from either the Lake Tahoe Basin Management Unit Office in South Lake Tahoe, or the Eldorado National Forest Ranger Station in Pollock Pines, or self-register after office hours.

Overnight backpackers can register for permits online at recreation.gov. Quotas are not in effect for the winter season. A $6 nonrefundable fee is required for each permit and additional charges include $5 per person for the first night and $10 for two to fourteen nights. Annual passes are also available for $20. Consult the website for more information.

Mokelumne, Granite Chief, and Mount Rose Wilderness Areas: Permits are not required at this time for winter use.

California Sno-Park Permits
For many years the State of California has utilized the SNO-PARK program to provide vehicle parking and access to popular winter recreational areas from November 1 to May 30. Day permits cost $5 and a season pass is $25. Permits can be purchased online at www.ohv.parks.ca.gov and then received in the mail (a temporary permit can be downloaded for printing at time of purchase). Along with parking space, SNO-PARKs include sanitation facilities, usually port-a-potties. Overnight camping outside of a vehicle is prohibited. Vehicles parked illegally are subject to a minimum $94.50 fine. More information is available on the website. SNO-PARKs used in this guide in the Tahoe area are listed below:

Sno-Park	Trips	Information
Donner Summit	6–11	USFS 530-587-3558, www.fs.usda.gov/tahoe
Donner Memorial State Park	12	DMSP 530-582-7892, www.parks.ca.gov
Meiss Meadow	36–38	USFS 209-295-4251, www.fs.usda.gov/eldorado
Carson Pass	39	USFS 209-295-4251, www.fs.usda.gov/eldorado
Echo Lakes	40–41	USFS 530-573-2600, www.fs.usda.gov/ltbmu
Taylor Creek	44	USFS 530-573-2600, www.fs.usda.gov/ltbmu
Blackwood Canyon	49	USFS 530-573-2600, www.fs.usda.gov/ltbmu

Equipment
The early 1970s saw a significant change in the design and composition of snowshoes. Prior to this point, the typical snowshoe was constructed from raw materials of wood and leather. Names such as "bearpaw" and "beavertail"

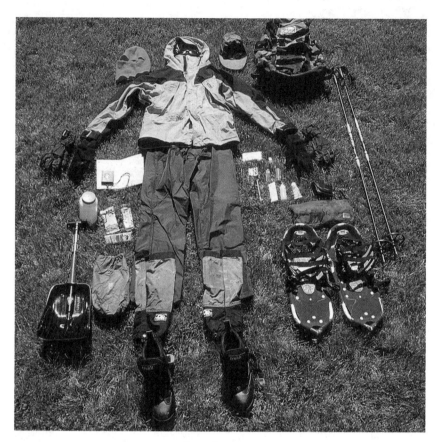

Snowshoe gear

described the shape of these oversized snowshoes, which required users to plod through the snow with altered strides and rangy motions. These shoes provided adequate flotation at the expense of large surface areas, forcing snowshoers to compensate by adopting gaits reminiscent of a cowboy walking away from his horse after a long day's ride. Nowadays, these old classics are more likely to be seen adorning the walls of rustic cabins or cafés than on the backcountry snow. Fortunately, modern-day snowshoers have much better snowshoes available for rent or purchase.

Snowshoes

Taking advantage of modern materials, new designs have revolutionized the sport of snowshoeing. Lightweight materials, space-age plastics, and advanced engineering have enabled designers to create lighter, smaller, and more efficient snowshoes. Rather than the cumbersome, oversized snowshoes of old, trim shoes with much improved bindings and traction devices have allowed recreationists to pursue winter trips with ease over a wider variety of terrain. High-angled slopes nearly impossible to navigate with traditional snowshoes are now commonly ascended without much difficulty with the newer, lighter equipment. The advanced design of snowshoes has definitely made the winter landscape more accessible by users of all skill levels.

Most modern snowshoes fall into the category of western, named for their origin in the mountain west. Developed for efficient travel over mountainous terrain, western snowshoes are generally smaller and lighter than their traditional counterparts. Shoes with both a tubular metal frame with a neoprene deck or a solid deck of molded plastic have found success in the marketplace. Advanced bindings are attached to the snowshoe usually with a single pivot point. Most have a crampon or traction device under the base for better purchase on hard pack or icy snow.

Manufacturers produce different types of snowshoes to cover the range of different snow conditions, but most users attempt to get by with a single pair. With some prices averaging well over $200, purchasing different sets for a variety of snow conditions would be a luxury to many. Some companies have overcome this cost barrier by providing interchangeable tails that can be attached to the main shoes in order to create more or less flotation to adapt to the broad spectrum of soft to hard snow. When purchasing a pair of snowshoes, make a choice that best fits the conditions you expect to encounter in the field.

Snowshoeing in the Sierra can present recreationists with a wide variety of snow types. Soft, fluffy powder is often encountered after cold winter storms, with snowfalls up to four feet not uncommon at the higher elevations. During such periods, enthusiasts likely desire the largest snowshoe they can strap to their feet. Once the snow becomes consolidated, users turn their attention toward smaller shoes with more maneuverability. During hard-pack conditions users want small shoes with good traction devices. The spring season presents perhaps the greatest shoe selection problem, when snow may be firm in the morning and mushy by afternoon.

Selecting the best snowshoe to cover all these possibilities can be daunting. Generally, try to get by with the smallest set of shoes that will reasonably handle the range of snow conditions likely to be encountered in the backcountry. If you plan to backpack, larger shoes will be necessary to accommodate the extra weight. If you're going to climb across steep terrain, lightweight, smaller shoes with good traction devices are preferable. When money is no object, buy as many shoes as needed to cover the spectrum of possible conditions. For the rest of us, carefully assess the likely conditions and make the best decision about one or possibly two pairs.

Poles

Poles are an important element in snowshoeing that some elect to forgo. However, they provide an extra measure of stability in keeping yourself upright. They also provide some exercise for the upper body and help to bear some of the load otherwise carried solely by the legs. Most snowshoe poles, as opposed to ski poles, are adjustable, which can be useful when snowshoeing over varying angled slopes. Some poles can be threaded together to form an avalanche probe.

Clothing

The backcountry rule of thumb for clothing is summed up in one word—layering. Many layers of lightweight clothing allow greater flexibility for adapting to the changing conditions often experienced when exercising strenuously in the winter. Adding or subtracting layers during changing conditions helps backcountry users regulate their body temperatures more easily than a few thick layers of clothing. Select base layers that utilize fabrics that wick away moisture and outer layers that are waterproof or water repellent.

Boots

Protecting feet from cold temperatures and the potentially wet conditions of winter is of the utmost importance. Many trips that start out as pleasant forays into the winter wonderland turn into living nightmares when feet become agonizingly wet and bitterly cold. Options for winter footwear have improved dramatically over the years and, with a proper fit, provide the foundation for more pleasant outcomes. A good pair of winter boots will help increase your odds of having a favorable trip. Some styles of winter boots on the market are better suited for snowshoeing than others.

When the weather is relatively warm and the snow not too deep, wearing waterproof hiking boots can be acceptable. If you choose this option, make sure your footwear is substantial enough to provide adequate support and comfort when attached to a pair of snowshoes. Fortunately, the Lake Tahoe area does not usually experience the number of bitterly cold days seen in other parts of the country, but your boots must still provide a moderate level of warmth. They should also keep your feet dry; particularly during spring trips when warm days turn the snowpack into wet mush by afternoon.

When selecting a pair of winter boots, make sure they provide the proper rigidity necessary for the successful operation of your snowshoes, as many winter boots might be designed for walking around in the snow but are not necessarily made for snowshoeing. Some models come with felt-type removable liners for extra protection from the cold—if you are considering purchasing such boots, make sure they fit well with or without the liners. Consult a trusted outdoor retailer for advice on purchasing the best set of boots for your needs.

Gaiters

A good pair of gaiters is essential for keeping snow out of your boots, thereby keeping your feet warm and dry. Select gaiters made from durable fabrics and that are easy to put on and take off.

Socks

Good socks are some of the most important pieces of winter clothing for keeping your feet warm. A wide variety of wool or synthetic socks are typically available from outdoor retailers. When wearing winter boots, the thickest socks are not usually necessary, as the boots should provide plenty of protection from the cold. Good-fitting socks should help to prevent blisters when paired with good-fitting boots.

Base Layers

A number of synthetic materials have been developed for use in the backcountry. Select base layers from fabrics well suited for conducting perspiration away from the skin and to the outer layers while maintaining the ability to keep you warm. While the majority of users go with synthetic fabrics, some still prefer wool or silk as the fabric of choice for their underwear. As nice as it may feel next to your skin, avoid cotton products altogether, as once cotton gets wet, you get cold.

Pants

Choose pants made from synthetic blends that are light- or mid-weight, water-resistant, and durable. Some users prefer loose-fitting pants for winter, while others prefer more tight-fitting pants. When the wind is blowing, or when it's raining or snowing, a pair of waterproof shell pants should go over your light- or mid-weight pants.

Tops

Modern fabrics have greatly aided the outdoor world in keeping winter users warm and dry. Multiple layers afford the ability to adjust to changing conditions, whether due to external or internal fluctuations in temperature. Pile, fleece, and other synthetic products provide a wide range of choices for what to wear on the upper body over the base layer. Shirts, vests, pullovers, and jackets can all be used alone or interchangeably to achieve maximum comfort.

When choosing layers, consider the advantages of down-filled products (high loft, lightweight, compressibility) versus synthetic-filled garments (retains loft when wet). When conditions dictate, the outermost layer should be a waterproof and breathable shell with hood.

Hats

In the Sierra you will most likely need a couple of hats. The first should protect from the intense rays of the sun on those idyllic, bluebird days. Baseball style or wide-brimmed hats are well suited for this purpose, as long as additional protection is provided for the neck and ears. The second should provide warmth when the weather is chilly or cold. A beanie or stocking hat is usually sufficient in the Sierra. When very cold conditions exist, a hat providing protection for the face may be necessary.

Gloves/Mitts

Along with cold feet, cold fingers and hands can make you miserable in the winter backcountry. Mitts will keep your hands warmer than gloves. Often the best combination is an inner glove liner made of synthetic fabrics and an outer shell made of waterproof fabrics with reinforced materials on the palms and underside of fingers. On warm days you likely will be more comfortable with lighter-weight gloves, such as cross-country ski gloves.

■ Safety Devices

Avalanche Transceivers

If you anticipate traveling extensively through areas of high avalanche potential, a transceiver would be a wise investment. To be effective, each member in your party must carry a unit and know how to use it effectively. Batteries should always be checked before each trip and an extra set carried in your backpack. For most low to moderate avalanche risk trips listed in this guide, transceivers should not be necessary.

Avalanche Probes

Probes aid in determining the location of avalanche victims. For most low to moderate avalanche risk trips listed in this guide, probes should not be necessary.

Snow Shovels

Carrying a snow shovel allows for digging out avalanche victims and can be used to build a temporary shelter if necessary.

Cell Phones

Although some parts of the Tahoe backcountry lack coverage, carrying a cell phone may provide a link to emergency services if they become necessary. Make sure phones are fully charged when embarking into the backcountry and either turn the phone off or minimize power use to conserve the battery in case you really need to call for help.

Personal Locators/Messengers

For areas without cell coverage, these electronic devices can be used to send a distress signal or communicate to the outside world in case of emergencies. They are not cheap and require a subscription but can be very effective when needed.

Navigational Aids

Snow cover is the most significant distinction of the Tahoe Sierra in winter when compared to the summer landscape. While hikers follow a well-defined path to their favorite destination during summer, winter travelers are governed by a much different set of circumstances. In the absence of defined trails, a modicum of navigational savvy is necessary to safely negotiate the snow-covered backcountry. Trail signs and tree blazes are lost, and even dominant physical characteristics, such as streams and lakes, can disappear or be significantly altered in appearance by the snowpack. In order to successfully negotiate the winter landscape, users must carry certain equipment and a working knowledge of its use.

GPS Units

With access to the GPS system by the general public, many outdoor lovers have become dependent on this technology for locating their position and getting to their destination and back again safely. Particularly in winter, when deepening snows obscure trails and landmarks, when competently used these devices can be a great asset in traveling safely through the backcountry. Since they are not completely reliable in all conditions, a GPS unit is no substitute for the ability to read a map and use a compass.

Map and Compass

A topographic map is essential when traveling through the mountains around Lake Tahoe. The gold standard for such maps is usually the 7.5-minute topographic maps published by the U.S. Geological Survey (USGS). These maps provide detailed topographic information with contour lines, elevations of important landmarks, and the location of important features, such as streams, lakes, mountains, and canyons. As with most tools, these maps are next to useless without a proper understanding. If you lack the ability to read these maps, you can acquire such skill through adult education courses or through an appropriate resource. USGS maps can be ordered through the USGS Store website (store.usgs.gov) for $8 per map plus shipping (2017). A number of apps have been developed to be used with smart phones as well.

In addition to the USGS maps, other valuable maps cover the Lake Tahoe area. The Forest Service publishes maps on waterproof paper for Desolation, Mokelumne, and Mount Rose Wilderness Areas at a scale adequate for backcountry travel. They also have maps for their ranger districts that lack topography and are too small for backcountry use, but they can be a fine aid for trip planning. Of the maps published by private companies, the Tom Harrison maps (tomharrisonmaps.com) are perhaps the best, with maps of Lake Tahoe and Desolation Wilderness available.

A detailed map covering your area of travel is essential but is incomplete without a properly working compass and the knowledge of its use. Avoid purchasing a cheap model—a flawed compass is worse than none at all. Poor visibility due to weather or terrain can disorient backcountry travelers and proper use of a compass is the best way to regain bearings.

■ Equipment Checklist

Essential Gear

- [ ] Snowshoes
- [ ] Poles
- [ ] Backpack
- [ ] Map
- [ ] Compass
- [ ] Headlamp or flashlight
- [ ] Knife or multitool
- [ ] Extra food
- [ ] Extra clothing
- [ ] Sunglasses and sunblock
- [ ] Matches and fire starter (in waterproof container)
- [ ] Candle
- [ ] First-aid/emergency kit
- [ ] Toilet paper
- [ ] Repair kit (cord, tape, safety pins, etc.)
- [ ] Water bottle or thermos (filled)
- [ ] Signaling device (whistle, mirror)

Optional Gear

- [ ] Camera
- [ ] Binoculars
- [ ] Sitting pad

Safety Equipment

- [ ] Avalanche probe
- [ ] Avalanche transceiver
- [ ] Cell phone
- [ ] GPS unit
- [ ] Personal locator/messenger
- [ ] Snow shovel

Clothing

☐ Boots	☐ Vest
☐ Gaiters	☐ Gloves and/or mitts
☐ Socks	☐ Hats (to protect against sun and
☐ Waterproof shell parka	cold)
☐ Waterproof pants	☐ Base layers
☐ Jacket	☐ Pants

▪ Snowshoeing and Nordic Skiing at Tahoe Resorts

North Tahoe

Squaw Valley offers snowshoeing and cross-country skiing in the meadow on the marked trail system at the Nordic Center near the Resort at Squaw Creek (call 530-583-6300 or visit www.squawalpine.com/events-things-do /snowshoeing for more information).

Northstar has a mid-elevation trail system through the Cross Country, Telemark and Snowshoe Center (call 530-562-3270 or visit http://www.northstarcalifornia.com/the-mountain/xc-snowshoe-telemark.aspx for more information).

Royal Gorge, North America's largest cross-country ski resort, also allows snowshoers on their routes and has snowshoe-only designated trails (www .royalgorge.com/snowshoe).

Tahoe Donner, just north of Truckee, has 100-plus kilometers of trails available to skiers and snowshoers, with 7.5 kilometers for snowshoers only (www.tahoedonner.com/cross-country/snowshoeing-trails).

Tahoe XC, located just north of Dollar Point, offers 65 kilometers of trail (www.tahoexc.org).

East Tahoe

Lake Tahoe Nevada State Park has had an on-again, off-again history with Nordic trails. At one time, a cross-country ski concession set tracks around Spooner Lake and up North Canyon to Spooner Lake, but less than adequate snowfall for more than one season made that enterprise unprofitable. More recently, a volunteer group named Nevada Nordic has been trying to get tracks set in the park.

South Tahoe

Hope Valley Outdoors operates out of a yurt near Picketts Junction. They rent equipment and groom tracks for 10 miles of trail (www.hopevalleycross country.com).

Kirkwood Cross Country Snowshoe Center offers 80 kilometers of machine-groomed trail, with skating and snowshoe lanes (www.kirkwood.com).

The Mountain Sports Center at **Camp Richardson** is the spot for winter recreation at the resort. Rentals of skis and snowshoes are available for use on their bike trails converted for winter use (camprichardson.com/recreation /winterspring-recreation).

(**Lake Tahoe Community College** has recently been grooming trails for skiers and snowshoers.)

◼ How to Use This Guide

This guide is designed specifically for snowshoers and cross-country skiers desiring opportunities for one-day trips into the Tahoe Sierra, an area centered around Lake Tahoe and roughly delineated by Interstate 80 in the north and California State Route 88 in the south. About 40 percent of the trips described are classified as moderate, 27 percent as easy, and 32 percent as strenuous. These ratings are subjective and prone to the random conditions of nature. A strenuous trip might easily be accomplished on a day when the weather is clear and the snow conditions perfect, while an easy half-mile trip could turn into a desperate struggle for snowshoers wading through five feet of fresh powder in a driving wind. The intention is that this guide will assist you in getting to the trailhead, to your chosen destination, and then back again with the minimum of difficulty.

The trip descriptions are organized into four parts: Part One, North Tahoe; Part Two, East Tahoe; Part Three, South Tahoe; and Part Four, West Tahoe. Each part begins with a short overview of the geographic area, main access roads, and major towns offering tourist services. After the overview, each trip description within a part contains pertinent information listed within several important headings.

LEVEL | This entry identifies the four levels of skill necessary to safely and enjoyably handle the trip—novice, intermediate, advanced, and extreme.

Novice trips require little, if any, experience, are essentially flat and short, and demand virtually no navigational skills. These trips should be able to be enjoyed by just about anyone, including children. Avalanche gear is not necessary at this level.

Intermediate trips will experience some elevation change and are generally longer than novice trips. Some navigation will be required to safely complete the route.

Advanced trips are longer, steeper, and more technically challenging than intermediate trips. They will require a higher degree of navigation as well. Snowshoeing experience is absolutely essential. These trips may present more objective dangers as well, such as higher avalanche potential, or a greater possibility of exposure to inclement weather.

The last rating, extreme, reflects trips pushing the limits of technical skill, endurance, and vulnerability to the forces of nature. These journeys are exclusively for advanced snowshoers who are technically proficient in all terrain, are in excellent physical condition, and are well qualified to evaluate potential hazards.

LENGTH | Accurate round-trip distances have been computed for each trip. Out-and-back trips start and end at the same trailhead. Shuttle trips start and end at different trailheads, requiring two vehicles, or being dropped off and picked up at two different locations. Loop trips start and end at the same trailhead but avoid much, if any, backtracking. Lollipop loops also begin and end at the same trailhead, but they have an out-and-back segment necessary to access the loop section.

TIME | The duration of a trip is listed here, based upon the amount of time necessary for the average snowshoer to complete the trip. People in excellent condition should be able to do these trips in a shorter amount of time, while less physically fit individuals will require more time than what is listed. Longer trips have been categorized into parts of a day rather than hours, which are more general evaluations and may also vary with one's level of physical fitness and the current snow conditions.

ELEVATION | The amount of elevation gain and loss appears under this heading. The elevation of out-and-back trips is listed as a one-way figure. Shuttle and loop trips are noted as round-trip figures.

DIFFICULTY | Divided into easy, moderate, strenuous, and very strenuous categories, this listing denotes the level of physical effort required to complete a trip. Easy trips should be able to be completed by just about anyone who is ambulatory, while very strenuous trips should be attempted only by people who are extremely physically fit.

AVALANCHE RISK | This category lists the degree of avalanche potential that may exist along the route in low, moderate, and high ratings. As conditions vary widely, this rating should not be taken as an absolute certainty but more as a general estimate of the terrain when the conditions for potential avalanches exist. Consult the current avalanche report (530-587-3558, extension 258, or www.sierraavalanchecenter.org) before venturing out into the backcountry.

DOGS | Many people wish to include their dogs on trips. In some areas dogs are not allowed, in others they must be on a leash. Where an OK appears, dogs are permitted off leash.

FACILITIES | Here is where you'll find a listing of any facilities near the trailhead, such as bathrooms, running water, and so on.

MAP | Pertinent maps appear here, which may be hard-copy maps available from retailers or maps that can be downloaded onto a computer from land agency or organizational websites.

MANAGEMENT | Government or, on occasion, private entities charged with the oversight of recreational lands appear under this heading, complete with contact information in case there are questions or concerns.

HIGHLIGHTS | Appearing under this heading are short listings of the main attractions for each trip, identifying the reason or reasons why this trip is worth your time and effort.

LOWLIGHTS | In contrast to the previous entry, this heading points out negative aspects, if any, that users should be aware of when contemplating a particular trip.

TIPS | Helpful information particular to trips is listed under this category.

TRAILHEAD COORDINATES | GPS coordinates are listed here for the trailhead for each trip. These waypoints are provided for your convenience. Some were checked in the field, but all were calculated using Google Earth. Use these waypoints at your own risk. Coordinates are no substitute for the ability to find your own way in the backcountry using navigational tools, such as an accurate topographic map, compass, personal GPS device, and the necessary route-finding skills. Waypoints beyond the trailhead have been omitted purposely, so users would not depend on them without the skills and equipment to find their own way in the backcountry.

TRAILHEAD | Accurate directions are provided for driving a vehicle to trailheads.

ROUTE | Accurate and detailed trip descriptions are found here.

MILESTONES | This section lists the major and significant points along the route with numbers corresponding to the accompanying map.

GO GREEN | For those who wish to give back their appreciation for our precious recreational resources, suggested activities or conservation organizations are featured under this heading, with the appropriate contact information.

OPTIONS | Additional routes or extensions are mentioned, as well as places to stay overnight in the backcountry.

WARM-UP | Many winter enthusiasts find a trip to the winter backcountry incomplete without sitting by the fire sipping their favorite winter beverage after an exhilarating romp through the snow. Some suggestions are provided for those who enjoy a hot drink or a warm meal following a snowshoe trip.

A completely subjective and random formula was used in evaluating these suggestions.

Trip	Duration	Distance	Elevation
Novice Trips			
8. Castle Valley Loop	½ Day	3.75	+600'–600'
12A. Snowshoe Adventure Trail	½ Day	2.9	Negligible
12B. Nature Trail	½ Day	1.8	Negligible
14. Tamarack Lake	½ Day	1	+200'–0'
23A. Spooner Lake	2 hours	2	Negligible
27. Big Meadow	2 hours	1.8	+350'–0'
30. Grass Lake Meadow	Varies	Varies	Negligible
40. Echo Lakes	Varies	Varies	Negligible
44. Fallen Leaf Lake	Varies	Varies	Negligible
45. Meeks Creek	½ Day	3.6	Negligible
46A. Yellow Trail	1 hour	1.2	Negligible
46B. Orange Trail	1 hour	1.2	Negligible
46C. Blue Trail	2 hours	2.1	Negligible
50. Page Meadows	½ Day	3	Negligible
Novice to Intermediate Trips			
20. Tahoe Meadows	Varies	Varies	+300'–300'
21. Chickadee Ridge	½ Day	3	+650'–0'
32. Grover Hot Springs State Park	Varies	Varies	+425'–0'
33. Hope Valley Overlook	¾ Day	5.8	+1,200'–275'
Intermediate Trips			
1. Pole Creek and Bradley Hut	Full Day	9.4	+1,800'–225'
4. Tahoe City to Cinder Cone	¾ Day	5	+1,250'–0'
6. Donner Lakes and Boreal Ridge Loop	½ Day	3.25	+750'–750'
7. Peter Grubb Hut and Round Valley	½ Day	5.4	+825'–150'
10. Andesite Peak	½ Day	3.6	+1,000'–0'
12C. Coldstream Trail	¾ Day	2.1	+250'–250'
13. Brockway Summit to Peak 7766	½ Day	1.25	+700'–0'
15. Fireplug	½ Day	1	+600'–0'
16. Galena Creek–Third Creek Loop	¾ Day	5.8	+850'–850'
17. Tamarack Peak	½ Day	3.2	+950'–0'
22. Tahoe Viewpoint Loop	½ Day	1.8	+275'–275'
23B. Marlette Lake	Full Day	9.6	+1,200'–350'
25. Castle Rock	½ Day	2.5	+275'–250'

Trip	Duration	Distance	Elevation
26. High Meadows	¾ Day	6.5	+1,400'–200'
28. Big Meadow to Scotts Lake	¾ Day	6	+900'–175'
29. Round Lake	¾ Day	6	+700'–675'
34. Hope Valley to Scotts Lake	½ Day	3	+875'–0'
35. Crater Lake	½ Day	3	+1,225'–0'
37. Meiss Lake	¾ Day	7	+400'–650'
38. Little Round Top	Full Day	10.5	+1,600'–500'
39. Winnemucca and Round Top Lakes	Full Day	6.5	+1,500'–1,500'
40. Echo Lakes	Varies	Varies	Negligible
43. Angora Lookout	½ Day	4	+650'–50'
43. Angora Lakes	Full Day	7	+875'–125'
46D. Red Trail	½ Day	3.3	Negligible
47. McKinney Lake	½ Day	7	+725'–775'
47. Miller Meadows	Full Day	12	+1,050'–775'

Intermediate to Advanced Trips

Trip	Duration	Distance	Elevation
3. Alpine Meadows to Five Lakes Basin	½ Day	3.4	+1,000'–0'
11. Summit Lake	½ Day	4.4	+300'–125'
41. Becker Peak	½ Day	3.4	+950'–0'
42. Ralston Peak	Full Day	5	+2,800'–100'

Advanced Trips

Trip	Duration	Distance	Elevation
2. Silver Peak	Full Day	9.6	+2,375'–0'
5. Donner Peak and Mount Judah	Full Day	4.6	+1,400'–200'
9. Castle Peak	Full Day	6.4	+1,900'–50'
12D. Schallenberger Ridge Loop	Full Day	10	+1,800'–1,800'
19. Relay Peak	Full Day	9.6	+1,400'–0'
24. Snow Valley Peak	Full Day	9.6	+ 2,450'–450'
26. Star Lake	Full Day	11	+2,650'–200'
36. Red Lake Peak	¾ Day	5	+1,500'–0'
37. Showers Lake	Full Day	11	+825'–700'
48. Buck Lake	¾ Day	10	+1,425'–275'
49. Stanford Rock	¾ Day	7	+2,200'–0'

Extreme Trips

Trip	Duration	Distance	Elevation
18. Mount Rose	Full Day	10	+2,100'–325'
31. Thompson Peak	¼ Day	1.6	+1,600'–0

Abbreviations

HTNF	Humboldt-Toiyabe National Forest
NDOW	Nevada Division of Wildlife
NSP	Nevada State Parks
SR	State Route
TRT	Tahoe Rim Trail
TRTA	Tahoe Rim Trail Association
USGS	United States Geological Survey
USFS	United States Forest Service

Legend

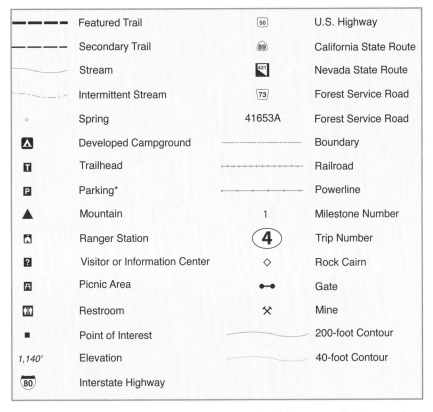

Symbol	Description	Symbol	Description
– – – –	Featured Trail	50	U.S. Highway
— — —	Secondary Trail	89	California State Route
	Stream	431	Nevada State Route
	Intermittent Stream	73	Forest Service Road
○	Spring	41653A	Forest Service Road
▲	Developed Campground		Boundary
T	Trailhead		Railroad
P	Parking*		Powerline
▲	Mountain	1	Milestone Number
	Ranger Station	4	Trip Number
?	Visitor or Information Center	◇	Rock Cairn
	Picnic Area	•–•	Gate
	Restroom	✕	Mine
■	Point of Interest		200-foot Contour
1,140'	Elevation		40-foot Contour
80	Interstate Highway		

* Numerous parking lots may be found on the maps. Trailhead directions will take you to the parking lot at the beginning of the trail of interest, indicated by a bold dotted line.

PART ONE

NORTH TAHOE

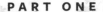

While the south side of the lake offers high mountain grandeur, the west side quiet serenity, and the east side undeveloped isolation, the north side combines elements of the other three. A wide variety of scenery and experience awaits snowshoers in the north part of Lake Tahoe's backcountry.

■ Access

The concrete ribbon of Interstate 80 provides indirect access to Lake Tahoe for the bulk of travelers heading to one of America's favorite winter playgrounds, and it's only fitting that the same highway serves as the gateway to many trips into the Tahoe backcountry. From I-80, three state highways radiate into the basin on the north side of the lake and provide access to trailheads.

Donner Summit is one of the easiest trans-Sierra passes in northern California to access, as the four-lane highway remains open all winter, except in the very worst winter conditions. A number of snowshoe trips begin at or near Donner Summit (I-80) and Donner Pass (old U.S. 40). With elevations over 7,000 feet, both passes attain altitudes usually sufficient to provide snowshoers with an adequate supply of snow for a lengthy season in average years. Frozen subalpine lakes, lofty summits, and beautiful vistas are here in abundance. Not only does the area offer visitors a wide range of scenery, but also plenty of trips for snowshoers of all levels and experience.

In addition to I-80, California State Routes 89 and 267 and Nevada State Route 431 provide additional access to trailheads for trips into the backcountry. Trips from CA 89 and CA 267 offer spectacular scenery and superb views. The Mount Rose Highway (S.R. 431) reaches its high point at 8,933 feet, the highest all-year pass in the Sierra, which provides high-elevation points of entry into the backcountry.

Although the north end of the lake has seen considerable development, the area doesn't feel as crowded as the south end. Nonetheless, a significant population of year-round residents coupled with part-timers and an influx of tourists can crowd some of the routes on a sunny winter weekend. If traveling from the west to Lake Tahoe, timing your departure to avoid the late Sunday afternoon crush of vehicles heading back to the Sacramento Valley or Bay Area should be a strong consideration. With a little planning, avoiding the crowds on the trail and on the highway is possible.

■ Communities

Major towns at the north end of Lake Tahoe providing visitor amenities include Truckee (airport, Amtrak station, Greyhound station), Tahoe City, Kings Beach, and Incline Village.

1 Pole Creek and Bradley Hut

The journey to Bradley Hut can be a pleasant experience, even for snowshoers and skiers not planning on staying overnight. Following a mildly to moderately graded road, travelers weave through a light forest for the first couple of miles and then follow the banks of Pole Creek another three miles into a scenic basin at the head of the canyon. Along the way are stunning views of 8,424-foot-high Silver Peak. With advanced reservations, the hut offers a fine base camp from which to explore the sloping terrain above the creek or the backcountry beyond (see Options).

LEVEL	Intermediate
LENGTH	9.4 miles, out and back
TIME	Full day
ELEVATION	+1,800'–225'
DIFFICULTY	Moderate
AVALANCHE RISK	Low
DOGS	OK
FACILITIES	None
MAPS	USGS *Tahoe City, Granite Chief*
MANAGEMENT	Lake Tahoe Basin Management Unit at 530-543-2600, www.fs.usda.gov/ltbmu
HIGHLIGHTS	History, overnight option, stream
LOWLIGHT	Limited parking

TIP | Beware of avalanche danger in the upper basin.

TRAILHEAD | 39°14.175'N, 120°12.441'W The trailhead is located along the shoulder of California State Route 89, 5.9 miles south of the junction of Interstate 80. A small plowed area on the west side of the highway offers limited parking, which is just south of Pole Creek and across from a wood house with a sign for OLSON CONST. CO. From the plowed area you should be able to discern the start of the snow-covered road, Forest Road 5708, paralleling the highway as it heads south into the forest.

ROUTE | [1] Follow the road on a winding climb away from the highway through moderate forest cover. Those who feel comfortable leaving the security of the road can save some time by traveling directly cross-country, rather than follow the circuitous route of the road. As the mild climb along the road continues, there are nice views of the surrounding hills and eventually Silver Peak. Around 1.75 miles, you reach a junction [2] with another road on the left, which heads toward Silver Peak (see Trip 2).

At the junction, you follow the right-hand road and head north on a moderate descent into the drainage of Pole Creek. Drawing near the stream, proceed up the gently graded road to a wooden bridge [3], cross the bridge, and then start a moderate climb above the north bank of the creek through widely scattered ponderosa pines. Along the way, the top of Silver Peak peers above the tops of the trees to the southwest. Around 3 miles, the road climbs more steeply and switchbacks up the hillside, reaching a junction [4] after one-quarter mile.

Veer sharply left at the junction and head west on a steady ascent. Stately Silver Peak makes regular appearances over the next mile above a widely scattered forest. After 0.9 mile, you reach an opening in the forest where the USGS map shows a road junction. Chances are you will not notice this obscure junction [5] when snow covers the landscape. Continue ahead (west),

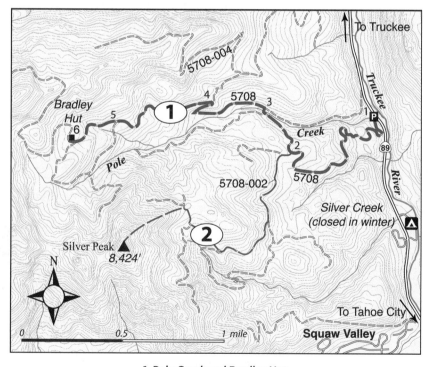

1. Pole Creek and Bradley Hut

crossing over a tributary channel and working your way west toward the upper basin. After .25 miles, the road curves left to follow a horseshoe bend. Just after where the road turns north, you find the relocated Bradley Hut [6] (39°14.012'N, 120°15.316'W) near the road on the fringe of the open terrain at the head of the canyon. *Note: just before the hut is another obscure junction with a road heading southwest toward Pole Creek—if you see this road, do not go in that direction.*

The two-story, A-frame hut with matching outhouse provides temporary shelter for day-trippers and accommodations for overnighters with reservations. The hut is equipped with wood-burning stove, tables, and kitchen. The upstairs loft can sleep up to fifteen people. When visiting the cabin, observe the posted rules and do your part to help ensure this historic legacy will continue for future generations. When your visit is over, retrace your steps back to the trailhead [1].

MILESTONES

1: Start at trailhead; 2: Turn right at junction; 3: Cross wooden bridge; 4: Turn left at junction; 5: Straight ahead at obscure junction; 6: Bradley Hut; 1: Return to trailhead.

GO GREEN | You can assist the Lake Tahoe Basin Management Unit by volunteering for short-term or seasonal projects. For more information, visit

---

HAROLD T. BRADLEY A university professor and former president of the Sierra Club, Harold T. Bradley, after experiencing the pleasures of the renowned hut system in the Swiss Alps, proposed a similar string of six alpine huts spanning the mountains above Lake Tahoe between Donner Pass and Echo Summit. Only four of the huts were ever realized, the last being completed in 1957 within Five Lakes Basin above Alpine Meadows. This final hut was named as a memorial to his late wife, Josephine.

In 1984, the inclusion of Five Lakes Basin within the designated Granite Chief Wilderness created a profound dilemma for the Bradley Hut, since Congress defined wilderness as "an area without permanent improvements or human habitation." After much debate, rather than simply destroying the structure, a plan was agreed upon to relocate the hut along Pole Creek. With the aid of many volunteers, the hut was relocated, refurbished, and reopened for the winter of 1998. Today, visitors can follow the record of the original construction and its eventual relocation through a photographic history on the walls inside the structure.

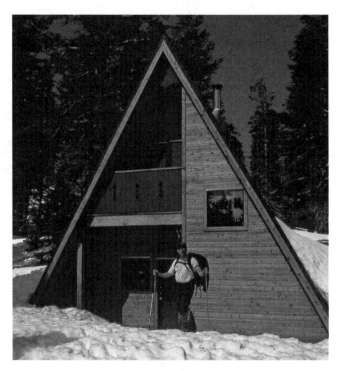

Bradley Hut

the volunteer page at http://www.fs.usda.gov/main/ltbmu/workingtogether/volunteering.

OPTIONS | For overnight reservations or more information about the Bradley Hut, contact the Sierra Club at Clair Tappaan Lodge (http://clairtappaan lodge.com). Hut reservations are accepted by phone (530-426-3632 from 9:00 AM to 5:00 PM) or by email (reservations@clairtappaanlodge.com). The lodge's mailing address is PO Box 36, Norden, CA 95724.

WARM-UP | When the "PIZ" fell off the sign out front, the owner seized the moment and renamed the restaurant ZA's. The momentous occasion aside, good food (appetizers, salads, pizza, pasta, and a handful of large plates) served at reasonable prices (at least by Tahoe standards) probably has more to do with their success than the offbeat name. Space is limited, so you may have to wait for a table, but you more than likely won't be disappointed by the food when it arrives—just don't be in a hurry. You shouldn't be too disappointed by the size of the check, either. ZA's is open for dinner seven days a week from 5:00 to 9:00. They also offer a Sunday brunch from 10:00 AM to 3:00 PM. Find the restaurant in Tahoe City at 395 Lake Tahoe Boulevard (Highway 28) across from the fire station and behind Pete and Peters, a popular watering hole. Call 530-583-9292 or check out their website at www.zastahoe.com.

TRIP

2 Silver Peak

During clear and sunny weather, Silver Peak provides one of the best lake views in the entire Tahoe Basin. Most of the trip follows a gently graded snow-covered road, but the last three-quarter-mile gains 1,000 feet up the northeast ridge to the top of the mountain, a steep ascent that should be attempted by experienced parties only. The lofty summit is quite airy and wind-prone—not the place to be when conditions are unfavorable. For those up to the task, Silver Peak rewards successful summiteers with an unsurpassed vista, which seems especially fine on sunny and windless days.

LEVEL	Advanced
LENGTH	9.6 miles, out and back
TIME	Full day
ELEVATION	+2,375'–0'
DIFFICULTY	Moderate to strenuous
AVALANCHE RISK	Moderate
DOGS	OK
FACILITIES	None
MAP	USGS *Tahoe City*
MANAGEMENT	Lake Tahoe Basin Management Unit at 530-543-2600, www.fs.usda.gov/ltbmu
HIGHLIGHTS	Summit, views
LOWLIGHT	Limited parking

TIP | For backcountry skiers and snowboarders, the descent of Silver Peak can be thrilling during stable conditions. Consult the avalanche report prior to your trip (sierraavalanchecenter.org).

TRAILHEAD | 39°14.175'N, 120°12.441'W The trailhead is located along the shoulder of California State Route 89, 5.9 miles south of the junction of Interstate 80. A small plowed area on the west side of the highway offers limited parking, which is just south of Pole Creek and across from a wood house with a sign for OLSON CONST. CO. From the plowed area you should be able to discern the start of the snow-covered road, Forest Road 5708, paralleling the highway as it heads south into the forest.

ROUTE | [1] Follow the road on a winding climb away from the highway through moderate forest cover. Those who feel comfortable leaving the security of the road can save some time by traveling directly cross-country, rather than follow the circuitous route of the road. As the mild climb along the road continues, there are nice views of the surrounding hills and eventually Silver Peak. Around 1.75 miles, you reach a junction [2] with another road on the right, which heads toward Pole Creek (see Trip 1).

Bear left at the junction and continue along the road headed south on a climb through a mixed forest of pines, firs, and an occasional incense cedar. If you want to forgo the road in favor of a more direct route, heading straight over Peak 7,403 to the northeast ridge of Silver Peak is possible. Otherwise, remain on the road as it arcs around a hill on a mild grade, reaching an overlook not quite 3 miles from the trailhead. From this vantage, you can gaze southwest over Lake Tahoe to Freel Peak, at 10,886 feet the highest summit in the Tahoe Basin. Another three-quarter mile along the road leads to the northeast ridge of Silver Peak [3].

Leaving the gentle grade of the road behind, climb much more steeply up the ridge. As you gain elevation, follow a direct line southwest up the ridge to the summit, except where a pair of rock outcroppings is passed on the right. The final pitch just below the top is fairly steep and may be wind packed,

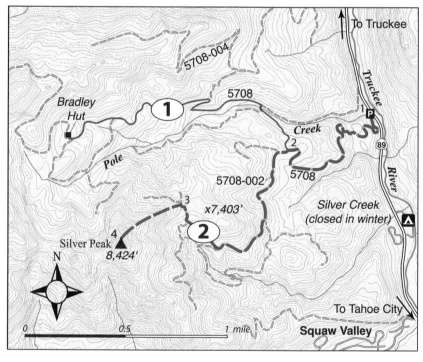

2. Silver Peak

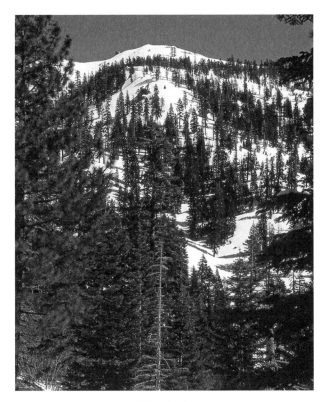
Silver Peak

which may require crampons and an ice axe to safely negotiate (39°13.228'N, 120°14.779'W).

The view from the summit [4] is spectacular, with Lake Tahoe revealed in all her glory and backdropped by a ring of peaks. Thousands of feet below, the busyness of Squaw Valley stands in stark contrast to the solitude at the summit. A fair amount of time can be spent watching brightly clad skiers and boarders descending the numerous runs. When the time comes, retrace your steps to the trailhead [1].

TRUCKEE RIVER Sixty-three streams flow into Lake Tahoe, but only one, the Truckee River, flows out of the big lake. The 121-mile-long river flows down the east flank of the Sierra Nevada, courses through the Reno-Sparks area, and eventually terminates in the Great Basin at Pyramid Lake, a remnant of ancient Lake Lahontan. The river, originally dubbed Salmon Trout River by John C. Fremont, was ultimately named for a Paiute chief who guided a party of emigrants to California.

1: Start at trailhead; 2: Turn left at junction; 3: Reach northeast ridge of Silver Peak; 4: Summit of Silver Peak; 1: Return to trailhead.

GO GREEN | Mountain Area Preservation is involved in protecting the greater Truckee area. For more information, go to their website at www.mapf.org.

OPTIONS | Silver Peak can be accessed on an alternate route directly from the upper parking area at Squaw Valley, providing you don't mind the typical congestion from one of Tahoe's premier resorts.

WARM-UPS | For an unbeatable start to the day, try one of the Squeeze In's numerous omelets at their narrow café in historic downtown Truckee (across from the train station at 10060 Donner Pass Road). The quirkily decorated restaurant serves breakfast and lunch from 7:00 AM to 2:00 PM daily. Call 530-587-9814 for more information.

3 Alpine Meadows to Five Lakes Basin

A short but strenuous climb leads to a quiet basin harboring five small lakes. An extremely popular summer hiking destination, Five Lakes Basin is lightly visited in the off-season. On a typical winter day, while hundreds, if not thousands, of skiers and boarders cavort along the nearby ridges and slopes of Alpine Meadows and Squaw Valley resorts, very few souls venture into neighboring Fives Lakes Basin. From the base of Alpine Meadows, a traverse across the steep mountainside past foreboding-looking cliffs and over to the lakes seems inconceivable at first glance. However, a passable route does exist for skilled snowshoers who don't mind the steep terrain. Due to the precipitous slopes and avalanche potential, experienced parties only should attempt this trip when snow conditions are stable and the ski resort is not involved in avalanche control procedures. The high, open terrain provides bird's-eye views of the stunning topography around Alpine Meadows during the ascent toward the basin.

LEVEL	Intermediate to advanced
LENGTH	3.4 miles, out and back
TIME	Half day
ELEVATION	+1,000'–0'
DIFFICULTY	Moderate to strenuous
AVALANCHE RISK	High
DOGS	OK
FACILITIES	None (ski resort nearby)
MAPS	USGS *Tahoe City*, *Granite Chief*
MANAGEMENT	Lake Tahoe Basin Management Unit at 530-543-2600, www.fs.usda.gov/ltbmu
HIGHLIGHTS	Lakes, views
LOWLIGHT	Limited parking

TIP | Consulting the avalanche report prior to your trip is essential (sierra avalanchecenter.org). The lower part of the route follows an easement across private property—please respect the rights of the landowners.

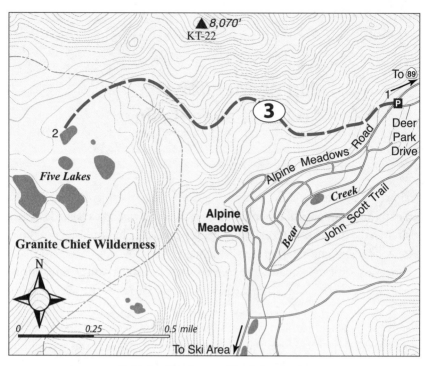

3. Alpine Meadows to Five Lakes Basin

TRAILHEAD | 39°10.759'N, 120°13.780'W Turn west onto Alpine Meadows Road, 9.5 miles from the State Route 89 off-ramp from Interstate 80, and proceed for 2.1 miles to the second of two intersections with Deer Park Drive. Park in the plowed area near the intersection—parking is extremely limited.

ROUTE | [1] Climb up the snow bank on the north side of the road and begin a moderately steep, continuous ascent across the south-facing hillside through a light covering of firs and pines. A cursory glance at the slope should reveal that this is not a place to be during unstable snow conditions, as avalanches occur here with some regularity and looming cornices appear on the ridge above. As you gain elevation, pleasant views of Alpine Meadows may calm your spirit where the trees begin to thin. During calm weather and good snow conditions, this slope is covered with myriad ski and snowboard tracks, which might further allay any apprehension. Continue the diagonal ascent across the north side of the canyon wall to a broad gully. Make an angling traverse around the head of this gully and then cross a ridge at the most convenient spot to avoid some rock cliffs. Once over the ridge, steady progress leads into another gully, where you should turn northwest and climb to its head. Ascend to the low point and then bear south across gentler terrain, where a short and easy ascent leads into Five Lakes Basin and the first of the lakes [2].

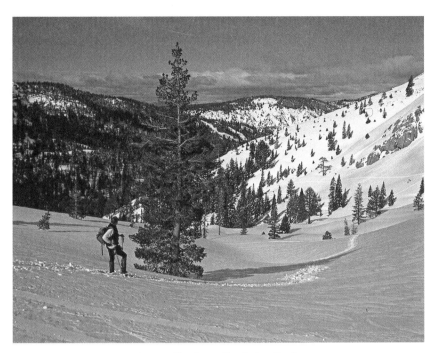

Descending from Five Lakes Basin

The relatively level, forested basin provides easy terrain for exploration of the other four frozen lakes if so desired.

MILESTONES

1: Start at trailhead; 2: First lake of Five Lakes; 1: Return to trailhead.

GO GREEN | Snowlands Network is a fine organization dedicated to protecting winter human-powered recreation across public lands. Consult their website at www.snowlands.org.

OPTIONS | While opportunities for further wanderings abound in the immediate area, please avoid the ski runs of Alpine Meadows.

RED FIR (*Abies magnifica*) Around where you enter the Granite Chief Wilderness, the upper montane forest transitions to a predominantly red fir forest. These conifers have adapted to the snowier and cooler climes above 7,500 feet. Mature red firs have longer cones compared to white firs, with dark reddish-brown bark. If you're unable to identify these two firs, try to twirl a needle between your thumb and index finger—if the needle rolls easily, it's a red fir, if not, then it's a white fir.

WARM-UPS | At the intersection of State Route 89 and Alpine Meadows Road, the historic **River Ranch Lodge** combines a roaring fireplace with a great view and good food. The restaurant provides a fine spot for a wonderful evening after a day in the snow. Disheveled snowshoers and backcountry skiers and boarders should feel right at home, despite the upscale dining and moderately expensive prices (dinner entrées range from $19 to $35). The full bar offers smaller plates for those searching for a less expensive option. Menus can be viewed and reservations made at www.riverranchlodge.com. The lodge also offers nineteen cozy rooms with mountain furnishings for overnighters (reservations strongly recommended).

On limited evenings during holiday weekends, Alpine Meadows offers a short, one-quarter-mile snowshoe tour to the mid-mountain **Chalet at Alpine Meadows** for a seated dinner from an Alps-inspired menu. Cost in 2017 was $69 per person. For reservations call 800-403-0206.

Tahoe City to Cinder Cone

For snowshoers who don't mind a nearly continuous climb with occasional steep sections, this trip from Tahoe City to Peak 7572 at the east end of the Cinder Cone provides supremely beautiful views of Lake Tahoe and the peaks rimming the basin. Nearly the entire lake's surface is visible from this northern vantage point, along with several ski areas, lakeshore communities, and other noteworthy peaks.

The first one-quarter mile is the steepest part of the climb, which leads to an open hillside with a fine lake view and a large wooden cross rising out of the snow—a memorial to a colorful former resident of Tahoe City. Most of the route travels through light forest, which inhibits the views until you reach the stunning climax at the summit. However, along the way are brief views of the lake, as well as Squaw Valley and Alpine Meadows ski areas.

LEVEL	Intermediate
LENGTH	5 miles, out and back
TIME	Three-quarter day
ELEVATION	+1,250'–0'
DIFFICULTY	Moderate to strenuous
AVALANCHE RISK	Moderate
DOGS	OK
FACILITIES	None
MAP	USGS *Tahoe City*
MANAGEMENT	Lake Tahoe Basin Management Unit at 530-543-2600, www.fs.usda.gov/ltbmu
HIGHLIGHT	Views
LOWLIGHT	Snowmobiles

TIP | Snowmobiles may be seen and heard in this area, with the highest chance of an encounter near a crossing of the Fiberboard Freeway at 1.75 miles, a major route between State Route 89 in Tahoe City and Highway 267 at Brockway Summit. Traveling on weekdays may minimize the chance of an encounter.

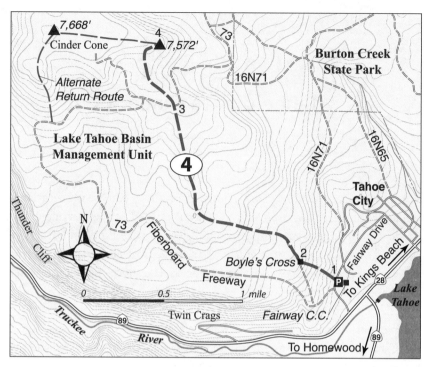

4. Tahoe City to Cinder Cone

TRAILHEAD | 39°10.153'N, 120°08.919'W At 0.2 miles north of the Y-intersection of Highways 28 and 89 in Tahoe City, turn east onto Fairway Drive. Follow Fairway for another 0.2 mile to the parking lot for the Fairway Community Center on the right. Park in the lot as space allows.

ROUTE | [1] Head steeply up the hillside opposite the community center across from the signed Tahoe Rim Trailhead and head northwest through a light, mixed forest of Jeffrey pines, white firs, sugar pines, and incense cedars. After one-quarter mile the terrain eases considerably near an old wooden cross sticking out of the snow (Boyle's Cross) [2].

Shortly beyond the cross, pass beneath a set of power lines and emerge from the forest into a pair of clearings. Beyond the second clearing, you head back into the trees and climb moderately up the slope. Eventually, the grade eases to more of a mild ascent. At 1.2 miles, the route veers north to follow a defined ridge, where the trees part on occasion to allow views to the west of the terrain around Alpine Meadows and Squaw Valley ski resorts. Continue along the ridge to a crossing of the so-called Fiberboard Freeway [3], 1.75 miles from the trailhead. In summer, the road is a sedan-worthy route popular with the mountain bike crowd but in winter is often used by snowmobilers, as evidenced by the preponderance of tracks you're likely to see here.

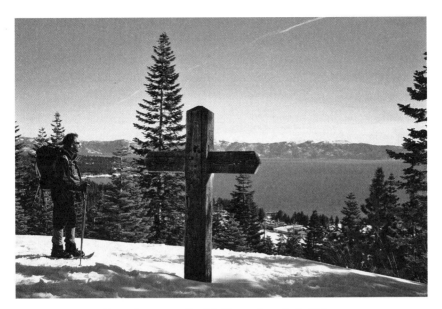

Snowshoer near Boyle's Cross above Lake Tahoe

Beyond the road crossing, climb the ridge northwest and then north toward Peak 7572. Nearing the top you curve east to arrive at an open, rocky aerie with an excellent view of Lake Tahoe [4]. Thanks to the exposure to the sun, you may be able to find a snow-free rock to sit on and enjoy the scenery. Nearly the entire lake is in view, rimmed by myriad snowcapped peaks. Numerous Tahoe landmarks appear around the basin—make sure you pack along a map for identifying them. After thoroughly enjoying the view, retrace your steps to the trailhead [1].

MILESTONES

1: Start at trailhead; 2: Wooden cross; 3: Cross Fiberboard Freeway; 4: Viewpoint; 1: Return to trailhead.

GO GREEN | Keep Tahoe Blue has been active at Lake Tahoe for sixty years, advocating, educating, and collaborating to protect the quality of the lake's environment. Consult their website at www.keeptahoeblue.org.

> **BOYLE'S CROSS** The memorial cross was placed sometime after long-time Tahoe City resident William Boyle was buried here on February 12, 1912. Legend indicates Boyle requested his drinking buddies bury him on this hill so he could continue to keep an eye on them. The spot is definitely a fine site for a memorial with a great view of Lake Tahoe.

OPTIONS | With the necessary route-finding abilities, you can avoid simply backtracking to the trailhead by heading west from the summit of Peak 7572 for three-quarters of a mile to Peak 7668 and then going generally south to intersect Forest Road 73 (Fiberboard Freeway). From there, simply follow the road back toward the Fairway Community Center.

WARM-UPS | The family-owned Fire Sign Café in Tahoe City has been a local hot spot since 1978. Extremely busy on weekends, the restaurant's freshly prepared dishes are worth the wait for either breakfast or lunch. Not only can you find the traditional bacon and eggs breakfast but more exotic fare like the Cape Cod Benedict or the smoked salmon omelette. Lunch and breakfast are served all day from 7:00 AM until 3:00 PM. The café occupies an old house at 1785 W. Lake Boulevard. Check out their website at www.firesigncafe.com for more information.

<table>
<tr><td>TRIP</td><td rowspan="2"></td></tr>
</table>

TRIP 5 | Donner Peak and Mount Judah

Two peaks with superb views are the primary rewards of this trip in the Donner Pass area. Although the overall distance is minimal, the climb is fairly steep, except for the broad ridge leading to the summit of Mount Judah. The slopes are a tad steep for most cross-country skiers, but backcountry skiers and boarders often careen down the north-facing slopes when powder conditions prevail.

LEVEL	Advanced
LENGTH	4.6 miles, out and back
TIME	Full day
ELEVATION	+1,400'−200'
DIFFICULTY	Strenuous
AVALANCHE RISK	Moderate
DOGS	OK
FACILITIES	None
MAP	USGS *Norden*
MANAGEMENT	Tahoe National Forest at 530-587-3558, www.fs.usda.gov/tahoe
HIGHLIGHTS	Summit, views
LOWLIGHT	No parking at trailhead

TIP | Avoid the corniced west ridge of Mount Judah.

TRAILHEAD | 39°19.065'N, 120°19.827'W From Interstate 80, take the Soda Springs/Norden Exit 174 and travel 3.6 miles east on Donner Pass Road to the Donner Ski Ranch parking lot. During periods of pleasant weather, you can also access the trailhead by heading up Old Highway 40 from Donner Lake.

ROUTE | [1] From the parking lot, walk along Donner Pass Road for 0.1 mile to Donner Pass and the start of the route near Sugar Bowl Academy. [2] Head down a snow-covered section of Old Donner Pass Road until you reach a convenient spot from which to head southeast up the moderately steep hillside of Donner Peak. Proceed up the mountain through widely scattered conifers, enjoying fine views of Summit Valley to the west and the peaks around Donner

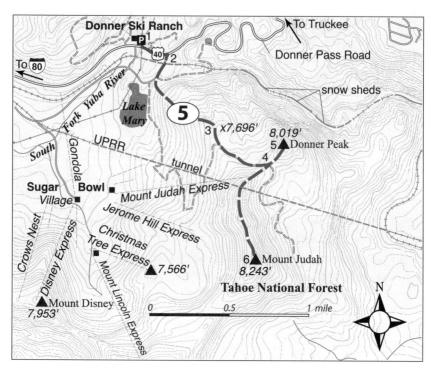

5. Donner Peak and Mount Judah

Summit to the north. Before actually gaining the top of Donner Peak, you must climb over a minor summit [3] (shown as Peak 7696 on the USGS map), from where you have a foretaste of the view awaiting at the true summit. Continuing the climb, pass through a stand of trees on the way to a saddle [4] separating Donner Peak and Mount Judah. From the saddle, turn northeast and make the short ascent up moderately angled slopes to the base of the summit rocks of Donner Peak [5]. Reaching the actual summit will require skills beyond the abilities of most. However, from the base there are marvelous views in all directions: Donner Lake lies at your feet to the east, while massive cornices oftentimes loom along the ridge of Mount Judah, and an array of peaks spreads out to the north and south.

Whether continuing toward Mount Judah or returning to the trailhead, retrace your steps back to the saddle [4]. From there, if satisfied with the trip to Donner Peak, retrace your steps back to the parking lot [1]. Otherwise, begin a steep climb southwest up the hillside toward the long summit ridge of Mount Judah, aiming for a pair of reflectorized signs at the north end of the ridge. Upon gaining the crest, the grade eases considerably on the way toward the true summit near the south end of the ridge. Continue along the crest while avoiding the cornices on the west side. After a slight dip, make the final easy climb to the top of Mount Judah [6].

Both the long ridge and the summit of Mount Judah offer a grand panorama of the north Tahoe countryside. A flurry of activity is usually ongoing on the slopes of Sugar Bowl and Donner Ranch ski areas to the north. Trains can often be seen chugging up the grade toward Donner Pass, while hundreds of cars snake along Interstate 80. The bustling community of Truckee spreads out in the east beyond Donner Lake. A more remote feeling occurs when looking to the south, where myriad snow-covered peaks stretch along the Sierra Crest, beckoning the adventurous toward further explorations. For most, the view from Mount Judah is sufficient, a fine reward for the journey. After thoroughly enjoying the scenery, follow your steps back to the car [1].

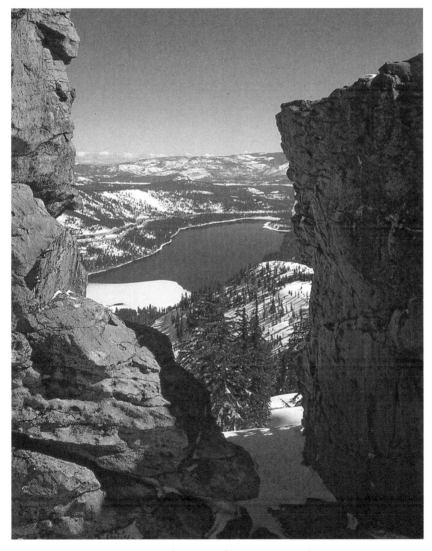

Donner Lake as seen from Donner Peak

THEODORE JUDAH Mount Judah was named for the railroad engineer Theodore Judah (1826–1863), who surveyed the route through the Sierra for the Transcontinental Railroad. He received the nickname "Crazy Judah" for such a bold idea of building a railroad through the difficult mountain terrain, a concept thought to be impossible at the time. Unable to raise funds for the project in San Francisco, he ultimately found success in Sacramento with the "Big Four" (Charles Crocker, Mark Hopkins, Collis P. Huntington, and Leland Stanford), who managed the financing and construction. He also was instrumental in helping to pass the Pacific Railroad Act in 1862, authorizing the project. Judah died at a young age after contracting yellow fever during a trip to Panama. The railroad was completed in 1869. The U.S. Board on Geographic Names affixed his name to the peak in 1940.

MILESTONES

1: Start at Donner Ski Ranch parking lot; 2: Turn right at Old Donner Pass Road near Sugar Bowl Academy; 3: Peak 7696; 4: Saddle; 5: Donner Peak; 4: Saddle; 6: Mount Judah; 1: Return to trailhead.

GO GREEN | Since 1987, Mountain Area Preservation has been helping to preserve the Truckee area's small town character and the natural environment. Consult their website at www.mapf.org.

OPTIONS | If you find yourself at the top of Mount Judah with plenty of extra time and energy, continuing along the Sierra crest southbound to Mount Lincoln or farther to Anderson Peak is possible.

WARM-UPS | A short (5.6 miles) drive east on Donner Pass Road leads to Donner Lake Kitchen (13720 Donner Pass Road), a family-owned café serving breakfast and lunch from 7:00 AM to 2:00 PM seven days a week. The huevos rancheros topped with chorizo is the house specialty.

TRIP
6

Donner Lakes
and Boreal Ridge Loop

Aside from the potential route-finding problems, this trip would garner an easy rating, as the distance is relatively short and the terrain is not particularly steep. However, the densely forested, undulating topography along the first mile may be confusing at times, requiring a modicum of navigational ability. For those willing to test such skills, the lakes offer pleasant scenery and Boreal Ridge offers fine views.

LEVEL	Intermediate 3.25 miles, loop
TIME	Half day
ELEVATION	+750'–750'
DIFFICULTY	Moderate
AVALANCHE RISK	Low to moderate
DOGS	OK
FACILITIES	Vault toilet
MAP	USGS *Norden*
MANAGEMENT	Tahoe National Forest at 530-587-3558, www.fs.usda.gov/tahoe
HIGHLIGHTS	Lakes, views
LOWLIGHT	Navigation

TIP | Avoid Boreal Ridge ski area by staying well to the east of the ski slopes.

TRAILHEAD | 39°20.380'N, 120°20.595'W Just west of Donner Summit, take Exit 176 from Interstate 80 signed CASTLE PEAK and BOREAL RIDGE RD. Follow signs to the SNO-PARK by heading east on the frontage road directly south of the freeway.

ROUTE | [1] From the east end of the SNO-PARK, head into moderate forest cover for a little over one-quarter mile on a course roughly paralleling the freeway. Near the edge of a clearing [2], turn southeast and head through mildly convoluted terrain to a hillside about three-quarters of a mile from the trailhead, where you should be able to spy Azalea Lake. Descend to the lake [3], which occupies a basin bounded by rock walls and steep hillsides.

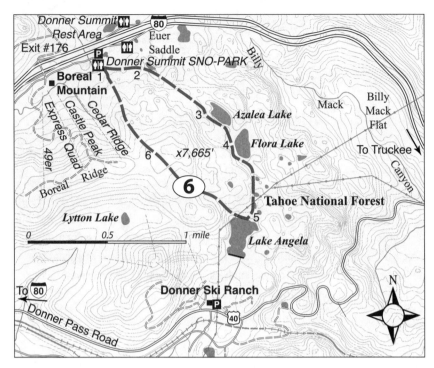

6. Donner Lakes and Boreal Ridge Loop

From Azalea Lake, head southeast through a narrow gap to Flora Lake [4], the environs creating a serene and picturesque setting well suited for a lingering break.

Heading away from Flora Lake, climb south directly over a less wooded rise, passing below a transmission line on the way to Lake Angela [5], largest of the three lakes on the circuit. The lake sprawls across the open terrain, allowing views of the Sierra crest peaks to the south of Donner Pass Road. Although quite scenic, the pristine nature of the area is otherwise compromised by the presence of the massive power line marring the north and west shores and the dam at the south end.

The next part of the loop begins at the northwest tip of Lake Angela, where a gully rises to the northwest up a hillside. Head up the gully on a moderate climb through light forest toward the crest of Boreal Ridge ahead. Aim for the top directly west of the easternmost high point (7665 on the USGS map) [6]. Attaining the ridge, you have marvelous views of the Donner Pass region.

From Boreal Ridge, descend into denser forest cover on the north side. Eventually, you should intersect your trail from the SNO-PARK, about three-quarters of a mile from the crest, where you turn west and follow it back to the trailhead [1].

1: Start at trailhead; 2: Turn right at edge of clearing; 3: Azalea Lake; 4: Flora Lake; 5: Lake Angela; 6: Top of Boreal Ridge; 1: Return to trailhead.

GO GREEN | The Northern Sierra Partnership is a collaborative effort that is involved in conserving natural areas in the northern Sierra, restoring the natural landscape, expanding recreational opportunities and education, and supporting local communities. Visit their website at www.northernsierra partnership.org.

OPTIONS | By leaving a second vehicle at Donner Ski Ranch, you could do a point-to-point route between Donner Summit and Donner Pass. However, this route would eliminate either the visit to the lakes, or the views from the top of Boreal Ridge.

WARM-UPS | Located in a shopping center on State Route 89 at the west edge of Truckee (11329 Deerfield Drive), family-owned Village Pizzeria will fill the bill for pizza or Italian specialties after a spin around the snow. You can see their menu at www.villagepizzeriatruckee.com and call ahead (530-587-7171) if you're pressed for time.

COYOTE (*Canis latrans*) Perhaps no wild animal has adapted to the urbanization of the American West better than this member of the dog family. Originally confined to the central United States and northern Mexico, coyotes have expanded their range all across the continent, due primarily to the near eradication of their chief competitor, the wolf. Ranging from 20 to 40 pounds, they are opportunistic hunters in the wild, surviving primarily on rabbits, rodents, and carrion. Coyotes close to urban areas will raid garbage cans and prey on cats and small dogs when available. In contrast to wolves, coyotes don't usually hunt in packs, preferring to hunt alone or with a mate. In urban settings, you're most likely to see an individual early in the morning or around sunset, whereas in the wild, they typically hunt during the day. In winter, coyotes grow a dense coat and secrete oils to help waterproof their fur. They also grow fur on their feet and between their toes for insulation and increased mobility over the snow.

Peter Grubb Hut and Round Valley

The convenient access and relatively short distance makes this trip popular with skiers and snowshoers alike. Due to such popularity, chances are you'll be able to follow a packed trail all the way to Round Valley unless you arrive immediately after a storm. An overnight stay at Peter Grubb Hut (reservations required) provides a reasonably comfortable way to explore some of the backcountry to the north, offering a degree of solitude that will almost certainly be lacking on the way to the hut. Clear days offer grand views of Castle Peak and the Donner Summit area from Castle Pass.

LEVEL	Intermediate
LENGTH	5.4 miles, out and back
TIME	Half day
ELEVATION	+825'–150'
DIFFICULTY	Moderate
AVALANCHE RISK	Low to moderate
DOGS	OK
FACILITIES	Vault toilet
MAP	USGS *Norden*
MANAGEMENT	Tahoe National Forest at 530-587-3558, www.fs.usda.gov/tahoe
HIGHLIGHTS	Hut, meadow, views
LOWLIGHT	Crowds

TIP | Parking closer to the start of the Castle Valley Road may be available on the north side of the Castle Peak exit from I-80, depending on current conditions and regulations.

TRAILHEAD | 39°20.380'N, 120°20.595'W Just west of Donner Summit, take Exit 176 from Interstate 80 signed CASTLE PEAK and BOREAL RIDGE RD. Follow signs to the SNO-PARK by heading east on the frontage road directly south of the freeway.

ROUTE | [1] From the SNO-PARK, walk along the access road to the underpass below the freeway and head to the north side and the start of Castle Valley Road [2]. Follow the snow-covered road, which soon turns northwest into mixed forest, where signs direct snowmobilers to the left and human-powered recreationists to the right. Continue along Castle Valley Road for a short while to the vicinity of Castle Meadow on the right. Excellent views of Castle Peak open up as you pass slightly above and west of the meadow and continue up the road on a mild grade.

Leaving the meadow behind, continue the gentle ascent toward the head of the canyon until a stiffer ascent delivers you to Castle Pass [3], where an

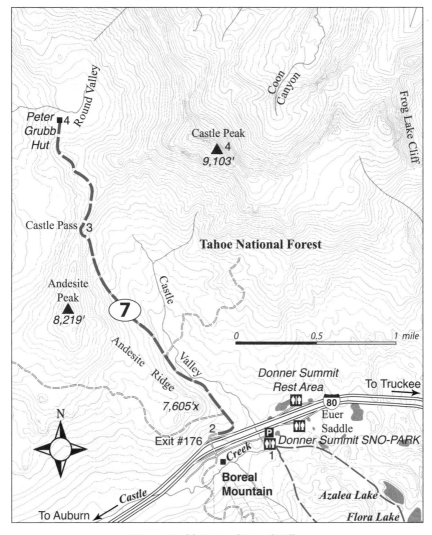

7. Peter Grubb Hut and Round Valley

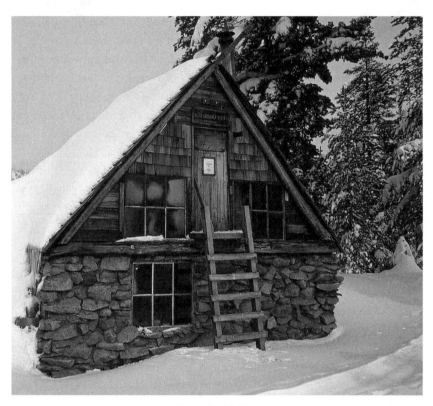

Peter Grubb Hut

excellent vista unfolds of the peaks of the Donner Summit region. The volcanic ramparts of Castle Peak loom directly above, while the ski runs of Northstar, Boreal Ridge, and Sugar Bowl carpet the nearby hills.

Avoiding the tendency to immediately descend the slope below the pass, continue on the ridge northeast toward Castle Peak, following some old orange, triangular markers signed SIERRA SKI WAY, CASTLE PEAK, and NORDEN. Eventually, your route leaves the ridge to make a gentle descent through light forest for a half mile to the edge of a hill overlooking lovely Round Meadow. A stiffer descent leads down to the meadow, where you can work your way over to Peter Grubb Hut [4] just beyond the southwest fringe (39°22.089'N, 120°22.053'W).

The hut makes a pleasant destination for a half-day outing, or a fine base camp for further explorations into the terrain beyond. The gentle, open slopes of Round Valley provide a fine environment for perfecting your technique.

When the visit is over, retrace your steps to the trailhead [1].

MILESTONES

1: Start at trailhead; 2: Start of Castle Valley Road; 3: Castle Pass; 4: Peter Grubb Hut; 1: Return to trailhead.

PETER GRUBB The hut was named as a memorial to Peter Grubb (1919–1937), who grew up in San Francisco and was an avid backcountry skier and mountaineer and a member of the Sierra Club. After graduating from high school, he sailed to Italy for a bicycle tour, where he died of an unspecified illness in Capri on October 21. Interested readers can read Peter's letters at http://clairtappaanlodge.com/peter-grubb-hut-history, which reveal his great love for the mountains. The hut is quite rustic but does provide a safe haven from the elements.

GO GREEN | You can support conservation of the north Tahoe region by joining the Sierra Club, either through the Toiyabe (sierraclub.org/toiyabe) or Mother Lode (sierraclub.org/mother-lode) Chapters.

OPTIONS | To spend a night or two at Peter Grubb Hut, contact the Sierra Club at Clair Tappaan Lodge (http://clairtappaanlodge.com). Hut reservations are accepted by phone (530-426-3632 from 9:00 AM to 5:00 PM) or by email (reservations@clairtappaanlodge.com). The lodge's mailing address is PO Box 36, Norden, CA 95724).

WARM-UPS | The Cottonwood Restaurant and Bar (10142 Rue Hilltop), located high on the hill just south of Truckee's historic downtown on the site of California's first ski jump, is a consensus winner for one of North Tahoe's top spots for dinner. One would hardly guess from the rustic appearance of the building's exterior that the ambiance inside of the establishment, while still maintaining the rustic theme, is warm and inviting. Executive Chef David Smith, has been here for nearly two decades and his menu features both local favorites and nightly specials. Be forewarned, some of the items on the menu are a bit pricey. Visit www.cottonwoodrestaurant.com for more information or to view a menu. Reservations can be made online or by calling 530-587-5711.

TRIP

8 Castle Valley Loop

Thanks to the 7,227-foot elevation and the dependable access via Interstate 80, Donner Summit provides winter visitors straightforward entry to some of the Sierra's best conditions. Weekends of fair weather will see plenty of skiers and boarders cavorting down the slopes of Boreal Ridge ski area, or more adventurous souls propelling themselves into the surrounding backcountry. While solitude may be a bit hard to come by in this area, plenty of potential destinations may allow backcountry users to disperse themselves around the region with some ease.

One of the least difficult routes in the Donner Summit area is the relatively easy jaunt around Castle Valley. Requiring only some gentle climbing

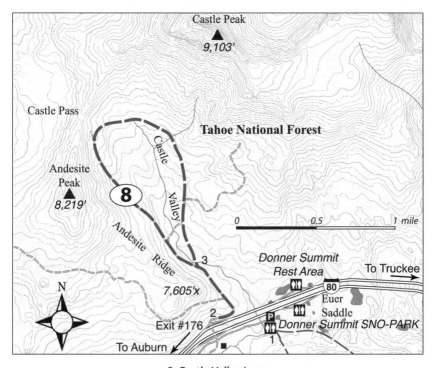

8. Castle Valley Loop

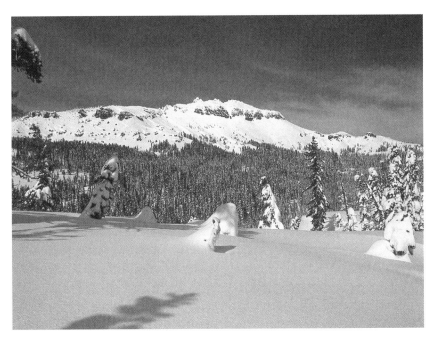

Castle Peak

and reasonably straightforward route finding, the less than 4-mile loop is well suited for novice snowshoers and skiers, while the beautiful scenery attracts more experienced users. Blue diamonds may aid in finding the way through forested sections of the route, but the configuration of Castle Valley should present few navigational difficulties. Views across the open meadow of Castle Peak can be quite dramatic.

LEVEL   Novice
LENGTH   3.75 miles, lollipop loop
TIME   Half day
ELEVATION   +600'–600'
DIFFICULTY   Easy
AVALANCHE RISK   Low
DOGS   OK
FACILITIES   Vault toilet
MANAGEMENT   Tahoe National Forest at 530-587-3558, www.fs.usda.gov/tahoe
HIGHLIGHTS   Meadow, views
LOWLIGHT   Crowds

TIP | Parking closer to the start of the Castle Valley Road may be available on the north side of the Castle Peak exit from I-80, depending on current conditions and regulations.

TRAILHEAD | 39°20.380'N, 120°20.595'W Just west of Donner Summit, take Exit 176 from Interstate 80 signed CASTLE PEAK and BOREAL RIDGE RD. Follow signs to the SNO-PARK by heading east on the frontage road directly south of the freeway.

ROUTE | [1] From the SNO-PARK, walk along the access road to the underpass below the freeway and head to the north side and the start of Castle Valley Road [2]. Follow the snow-covered road, which soon turns northwest into mixed forest, where signs direct snowmobilers to the left and human-powered recreationists to the right. Continue along Castle Valley Road for a short while to the vicinity of Castle Meadow on the right. Excellent views of Castle Peak open up as you pass slightly above and west of the meadow and continue up the road on a mild grade. Unless your trip coincides with the middle of a snowstorm, you should be able to follow the tracks of previous users on this very popular route. Otherwise, periodically placed blue markers nailed to trees may help to guide you.

Leaving the meadow behind, continue ascending mildly up the valley through light-to-moderate forest to the base of the hillside below Castle Pass. From there, follow a slightly descending traverse through the trees to the far side of the Castle Valley drainage. Continue the descent where the route bends south to follow the east side of the valley. Around 2.75 miles, you break out of the forest into meadows, traverse the clearing for a half mile, and then regain the Castle Valley Road at the close of the loop section [3]. From there, retrace your steps back to the parking area [1].

STELLER'S JAY (*Cyanocitta stelleri*) Perhaps the most conspicuous bird in the Sierra Nevada, due to its harsh cry and boldness, the Steller's Jay has a black head and upper body, and strikingly blue lower body and wings, and is the only crested jay west of the Rockies. While many birds migrate away from the cold winters at Tahoe, this jay is here year-round.

MILESTONES

1: Start at trailhead; 2: Start of Castle Valley Road; 3: Close of the loop section; 1: Return to trailhead.

WARM-UPS | Marty's Café, a block west of the train station in the old historic downtown of Truckee (10115 Donner Pass Road), is a sure-fire hit for comfort food done exquisitely for breakfast or lunch, served seven days a week. Visit their website at www.martyscafetruckee.com to check out the menu or for more information.

9 | Castle Peak

The rugged ramparts of Castle Peak dominate the landscape to the north of Donner Summit. At 9,103 feet high, they tower above the surrounding countryside and dwarf nearby peaks and ridges. Coveted by alpinists and ski-mountaineers alike, the climb to the top provides a stimulating challenge for those up to the task. The first couple of miles to Castle Pass are relatively mild, gaining less than 750 vertical feet, but the climb from the pass to the summit is an entirely different story, gaining 1,200 feet in a mere mile. Only skilled travelers comfortable with high-angle slopes should consider going beyond Castle Pass. Successful summiteers will enjoy stunning views of the north Tahoe landscape.

LEVEL	Advanced
LENGTH	6.4 miles, out and back
TIME	Full day
ELEVATION	+1,900'–50'
DIFFICULTY	Strenuous
AVALANCHE RISK	Moderate to high
DOGS	OK (not recommended beyond Castle Pass)
FACILITIES	Vault toilet
MAP	USGS *Norden*
MANAGEMENT	Tahoe National Forest at 530-587-3558, www.fs.usda.gov/tahoe
HIGHLIGHTS	Summit, views
LOWLIGHT	Crowds

TIP | Parking closer to the start of the Castle Valley Road may be available on the north side of the Castle Peak exit from I-80, depending on current conditions and regulations.

TRAILHEAD | 39°20.380'N, 120°20.595'W Just west of Donner Summit, take Exit 176 from Interstate 80 signed CASTLE PEAK and BOREAL RIDGE RD. Follow signs to the SNO-PARK by heading east on the frontage road directly south of the freeway.

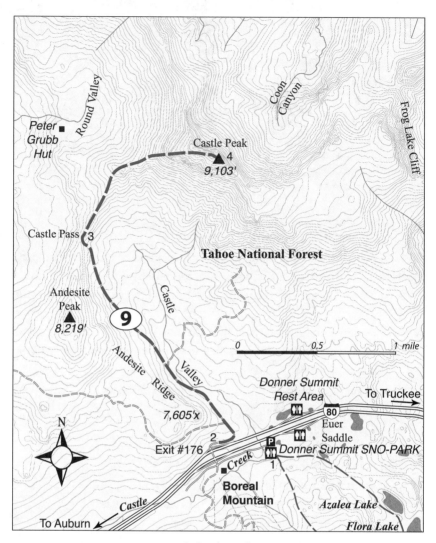

9. Castle Peak

ROUTE | [1] From the SNO-PARK, walk along the access road to the underpass below the freeway and head to the north side and the start of Castle Valley Road [2]. Follow the snow-covered road, which soon turns northwest into mixed forest, where signs direct snowmobilers to the left and human-powered recreationists to the right. Continue along Castle Valley Road for a short while to the vicinity of Castle Meadow on the right. Excellent views of Castle Peak open up as you pass slightly above and west of the meadow and continue up the road on a mild grade.

Leaving the meadow behind, continue the gentle ascent toward the head of the canyon until a stiffer ascent delivers you to Castle Pass [3], where an excellent vista unfolds of the peaks of the Donner Summit region. The volcanic ramparts of Castle Peak loom directly above, while the ski runs of Northstar, Boreal Ridge, and Sugar Bowl carpet the nearby hills.

From Castle Pass, head moderately steeply up the west ridge of Castle Peak. Higher up the ridge, bear slightly north of the ridgeline and follow less precipitous slopes toward the summit. Nearing the top, veer southeast and head for the top [4]. Depending on conditions, the last part of the ascent may be easier sans snowshoes, and the actual summit may be difficult to attain without mountaineering equipment and climbing skills. Even from just below the true summit, the view is remarkable, extending south to peaks above the far end of the lake and north to Sierra Buttes.

After thoroughly enjoying the vista, retrace your steps to the trailhead [1], or alter your return as noted in Options.

> CASTLE PEAK One glance at Castle Peak quickly reveals the origin of the name, as multiple rocky spires and ramparts line the summit ridge. Originally named Stanford Mountain by the Whitney Survey (1860–1864), the rock is primarily volcanic in nature.

MILESTONES

1: Start at trailhead; 2: Start of Castle Valley Road; 3: Castle Pass; 4: Castle Peak; 1: Return to trailhead.

GO GREEN | In 2016, the Truckee Donner Land Trust and the Trust for Public Land were instrumental in acquiring a 408-acre parcel north of I-80, which was turned over to the Forest Service. The parcel included the initial course of Castle Valley Road and a segment of the Pacific Crest Trail. You can learn more about the work of these two conservation organizations at www.tdland trust.org and www.tpl.org.

OPTIONS | Those who prefer to not simply retrace their steps back to the car can descend the southeast ridge of Castle Peak and then loop back to the trailhead with a bit of navigation.

WARM-UPS | Wild Cherries Coffee House (11429 Donner Pass Road), north of I-80 and one block west of CA 89, is a favorite among Truckee residents and visitors. In addition to the usual dose of caffeine, Wild Cherries has breakfast sandwiches in the morning and soups, salads, panini sandwiches, and other sandwiches for lunch. Visit their website at www.wildcherriescoffee house.com.

The ascent of Andesite Peak is a reasonably short trip to fantastic views of the northern realm of the Lake Tahoe area. The vistas are nearly as good as those from the summit of neighboring Castle Peak but require 3 fewer miles and 900 fewer vertical feet. Except for a couple of short, steep slopes, one near the beginning and one at the top of the peak, the trip would garner an easy rating, as the navigation is fairly straightforward—simply gain the ridge and follow it to the top. Once away from Castle Valley Road, you should see far fewer fellow travelers.

LEVEL	Intermediate
LENGTH	3.6 miles, out and back
TIME	Half day
ELEVATION	+1,000'–0'
DIFFICULTY	Moderate
AVALANCHE RISK	Low to moderate
DOGS	OK
FACILITIES	Vault toilet
MAP	USGS *Norden*
MANAGEMENT	Tahoe National Forest at 530-587-3558, www.fs.usda.gov/tahoe
HIGHLIGHTS	Summit, views
LOWLIGHT	Snowmobiles

TIP | Parking closer to the start of the Castle Valley Road may be available on the north side of the Castle Peak exit from I-80, depending on current conditions and regulations.

TRAILHEAD | 39°20.380'N, 120°20.595'W Just west of Donner Summit, take Exit 176 from Interstate 80 signed CASTLE PEAK and BOREAL RIDGE RD. Follow signs to the SNO-PARK by heading east on the frontage road directly south of the freeway.

ROUTE | [1] From the SNO-PARK, walk along the access road to the underpass below the freeway and head to the north side and the start of Castle Valley

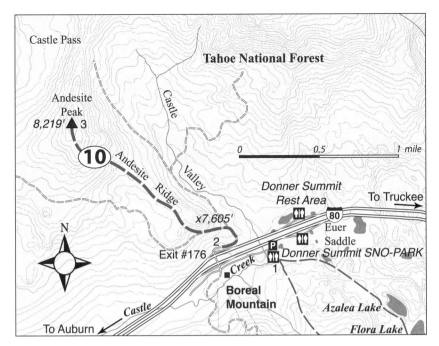

10. Andesite Peak

Road [2]. Follow the snow-covered road, which soon turns northwest into mixed forest, where signs direct snowmobilers to the left and human-powered recreationists to the right. Leave the road and head directly up a tree-covered slope below Andesite Ridge. After 0.1 mile you intersect a road heading west, which you follow for a short distance, and then find a convenient spot from which to begin a curving ascent of the steep slopes below Peak 7605 as shown on the USGS map. The immediate goal is the top of Andesite Ridge just below and north of Peak 7605.

Once at the top of the ridge, the grade eases considerably as you follow the ridge northwest. The scattered forest allows for sublime views of Castle Peak and the Donner Summit area, while straight ahead is the summit of Andesite Peak. An easy half mile of travel leads you back into the trees near the base of the summit. Staying away from the extreme east edge to avoid cornices, make a stiffer climb up the last 600 feet of the mountain, initially passing through heavy timber until the trees begin to thin and the views open up again higher up the peak. The terrain eases where you reach the final ridge leading to the broad summit of Andesite Peak [3].

The 360-degree view is quite spectacular: Castle Peak looms majestically to the immediate northwest, while off in the distance in all directions is an incredible panorama of north Tahoe peaks. When the time comes, retrace your steps back to the parking area [1].

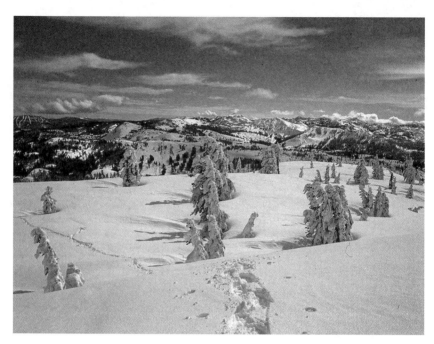

On top of Andesite Peak

MILESTONES

1: Start at trailhead; 2: Start of Castle Valley Road; 3: Andesite Peak; 1: Return to trailhead.

GO GREEN | In 2016, the Truckee Donner Land Trust and the Trust for Public Land were instrumental in acquiring a 408-acre parcel north of I-80, which was turned over to the Forest Service. The parcel included the initial course of Castle Valley Road and a segment of the Pacific Crest Trail. You can learn

WHITE FIR (*Abies concolor*) The most abundant conifer in the Tahoe Basin is the white fir, which can attain heights of 60 to 200 feet. A member of the upper montane forest, this evergreen is usually found in mixed forests, appearing with ponderosa pines, Jeffrey pines, western white pines, sugar pines, and incense cedars. At higher elevations, white firs may intermix with a close companion, red firs. Somewhat difficult to distinguish from each other, mature white firs have dark-gray, deeply furrowed bark and 2- to 5-inch-long cones. In contrast, red firs have dark-reddish-brown bark and 4- to 8-inch cones. If you're unable to identify these two firs, try to twirl a needle between your thumb and index finger—if the needle rolls easily, it's a red fir, if not, it's a white fir.

more about the work of these two conservation organizations at www.tdland trust.org and www.tpl.org.

OPTIONS | You could fairly easily extend and vary the return by descending the north ridge of Andesite Peak to Castle Pass and then following the Castle Valley Road back to the start.

WARM-UPS | Family-owned Morgan's Lobster Shack & Fish Market in downtown Truckee (10087 River St.) serves up some of the freshest East-coast style seafood dishes in the region, including Lobster Mac & Cheese, Lobster Rolls, and a Lobster Reuben. The establishment is small and often busy, but you shouldn't be disappointed with the food. Visit their website at www .morganslobstershack.com.

11 | Summit Lake

The trip to Summit Lake provides a pleasant alternative to the "freeway" of the Castle Valley Road routes. However, without a marked trail or road to follow, travelers will have to put their route-finding skills to the test in order to reach the lake and get back to the trailhead. Where the route passes through open terrain, there are some fine views of the Donner Summit region, and the secluded lake is a worthy destination for a half-day journey away from the crowds.

LEVEL	Intermediate to advanced
LENGTH	4.4 miles, out and back
TIME	Half day
ELEVATION	+300'–125'
DIFFICULTY	Moderate
AVALANCHE RISK	Low
DOGS	OK
FACILITIES	Vault toilet
MAP	USGS *Norden*
MANAGEMENT	Tahoe National Forest at 530-587-3558, www.fs.usda.gov/tahoe
HIGHLIGHTS	Lake, views
LOWLIGHT	Navigation

TIP | While an attractive option at first glance, you can't park at the westbound Donner Summit Rest Area off Interstate 80 and begin the trip from there (saving a mile), as parking for recreational purposes is not allowed and is subject to fines. Parking closer to the start of the Castle Valley Road may be available on the north side of the Castle Peak exit from I-80, depending on current conditions and regulations.

TRAILHEAD | 39°20.380'N, 120°20.595'W Just west of Donner Summit, take Exit 176 from Interstate 80 signed CASTLE PEAK and BOREAL RIDGE RD. Follow signs to the SNO-PARK by heading east on the frontage road directly south of the freeway.

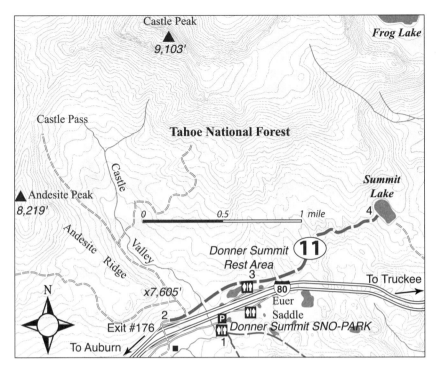

11. Summit Lake

ROUTE | [1] From the SNO-PARK, walk along the access road to the under-pass below the freeway and head to the north side and the start of Castle Valley Road [2]. Follow the snow-covered road, which soon turns northwest into mixed forest, where signs direct snowmobilers to the left and human-powered recreationists to the right. At this point, leave the road and head east-northeast, roughly paralleling Interstate 80. Cross the ravine draining Castle Valley and work your way over to the slope just above the westbound freeway rest area [3].

From above the vicinity of the rest area, head northeast, angling slightly away from the freeway. Although the overall route has minimal elevation gain, the topography is such that you must work your way over hummocks, across drainages, and around minor hills, continually negotiating minor elevation changes. Attempt to maintain a direct route by following a visual fix on a point at the end of the southeast ridge extending down from Castle Peak. Summit Lake nestles into a shallow basin just below the end of that ridge.

Unless the day is very windy and you desire the protection of the forest, you can set a course through mostly open terrain for much of the route to the lake. Away from the forest, you have marvelous views of Castle Peak with its towering ramparts and the greater Donner Summit region. The open views offer plenty of visible landmarks to aid in staying on track, such as Interstate

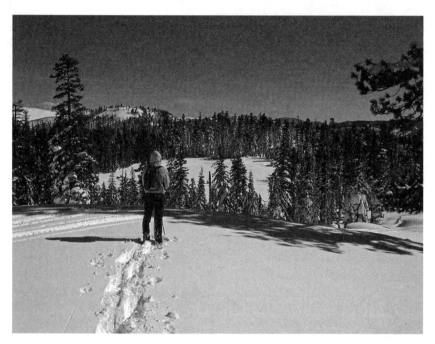

Snowshoer above Summit Lake

80 and Boreal Ridge ski area. On the final approach to the lake, the best route stays well above it, avoiding some steep terrain to the south plunging toward the freeway. Cross the crest of a ridge and drop to forest-rimmed Summit Lake [4]. The lake, pristine in appearance, offers a relatively tranquil atmosphere with the din of automobile traffic on Interstate 80 slightly audible.

BLACK BEAR (*Ursus americanus*) Black bears are common residents in the Sierra Nevada region, with an estimated population of 10,000 to 15,000 individuals. Despite the name, these omnivores can also be shades of brown, blonde, and cinnamon. Some males can reach up to 600 pounds, but the average size of adults is between 300 and 350 pounds. These fascinating mammals have rather poor eyesight, but their hearing is good and they have an excellent sense of smell. Black bears are very fast, attaining speeds up to 15 miles per hour. They are also good tree climbers. While many black bears will hibernate during cold and snowy winters, some will wake up and emerge from their dens periodically. In dry and warm years they may not hibernate at all, especially those who have adapted well to the urban interface. So, seeing one of these bruins on a snowshoe trip might be unusual but not impossible.

1: Start at trailhead; 2: Start of Castle Valley Road; 3: Veer slightly left near rest area; 4: Summit Lake; 1: Return to trailhead.

GO GREEN | In 2016, the Truckee Donner Land Trust and the Trust for Public Land were instrumental in acquiring a 408-acre parcel north of I-80, which was turned over to the Forest Service. The parcel included the initial course of Castle Valley Road and a segment of the Pacific Crest Trail. You can learn more about the work of these two conservation organizations at www.tdland trust.org and www.tpl.org.

OPTIONS | The terrain below Castle Peak certainly presents additional areas for further wanderings.

WARM-UPS | Moody's, in the historic Truckee Hotel (10007 Bridge Street), is a favorite bistro among locals and tourists, serving appetizers, soups and salads, pizzas, pastas, and entrées daily from 11:30 AM to 9:30 PM, with live music on the weekends. Check out their website at www.moodysbistro.com.

TRIP 12 Donner Memorial State Park Loops

The essentially flat landscape within Donner Memorial State Park is a great place for neophytes searching for some easy terrain to practice their ski or snowshoe technique. Five designated routes offer plenty of options for cross-country skiers and snowshoers. However, the trails may not be well marked, particularly following storms, as the park depends on volunteer labor for such tasks. Generally, the ski and snowshoe routes to Donner Lake see enough use that recreationists can follow the tracks of previous users. The less used routes (Nature Trail, Coldstream Trail, and Upper Coldstream Trail) will require some route-finding skill.

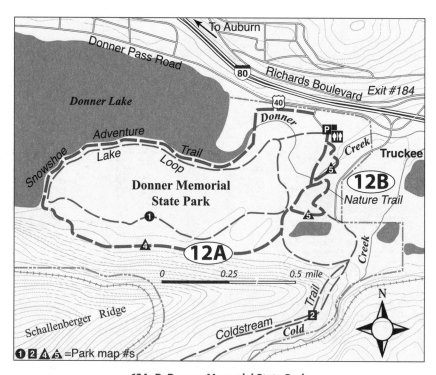

12A, B. Donner Memorial State Park

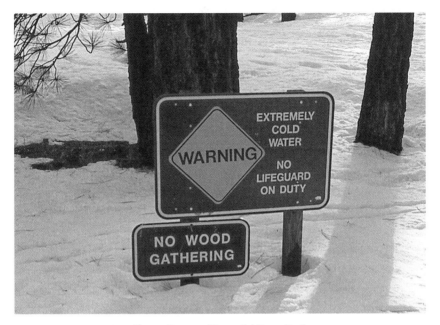

Sign at Donner Memorial State Park

Cross-country skiers and snowshoers can loop around the park on the popular 2.5-mile Lake Loop Trail, or the slightly longer 2.9-mile Snowshoe Adventure Trail. The gentle topography and short distance (1.8 mile) of the Nature Trail offers a safe and easy environment for families with children. Even for more advanced users, the park loops provide a fine place to spend part of a day serenely wandering through the scattered trees and catching glimpses of Donner Lake. The park also offers a 2.1-mile loop on the Coldstream Trail and access to Forest Service backcountry beyond on the Upper Coldstream Trail. As always, snowshoers are advised to stay out of fresh ski tracks. Incorporating a visit to the Emigrant Trail Museum would be an added treat, and, with a location just outside Truckee, a hot beverage or a warm meal at one of the many fine establishments would cap off an excellent day in the snow.

TIP | With an elevation slightly below 6,000 feet, you should check the snow and weather conditions before your visit to the park.

TRAILHEAD | 39°19.439'N, 120°13.966'W From Interstate 80, take Exit 184 signed for Donner Pass Road. At the four-way stop, turn right and follow Donner Pass Road for 0.3 mile to a left-hand turn into Donner Memorial State Park. For the Lake Loop and Snowshoe Adventure Trails, follow the park access road to the parking lot near the entrance station. For the Nature and Coldstream Trails, turn left and park near the museum.

LEVEL	Novice
LENGTH	2.9 miles, loop
TIME	Half day
ELEVATION	Negligible
DIFFICULTY	Easy
AVALANCHE RISK	Low
DOGS	Not allowed
FACILITIES	Museum, picnic areas, ranger station, restrooms
MAP	*Donner Memorial State Park Winter Trail Map* (web map)
MANAGEMENT	California State Parks at 530-582-7892, www.parks.ca.gov
HIGHLIGHTS	Child-friendly, forest, history, lake
LOWLIGHT	Low elevation

ROUTE | Find the start of the Snowshoe Adventure Trail on the west side of the parking area and head generally north-northwest to where the route bends south, crosses Donner Creek on a wooden bridge, and then follows a counterclockwise circuit through the park, initially following the shoreline of Donner Lake. After about a mile, bend away from the lake near the west end and head eastbound through light forest for another mile or so, reaching a junction with Coldstream Trail #2. Head northeast and continue back to the parking lot.

LEVEL	Novice
LENGTH	1.8 miles, loop
TIME	Half day
ELEVATION	Negligible
DIFFICULTY	Easy
AVALANCHE RISK	Low
DOGS	Not allowed
FACILITIES	Museum, picnic areas, ranger station, restrooms
MAP	*Donner Memorial State Park Winter Trail Map* (web map)
MANAGEMENT	California State Parks at 530-582-7892, www.parks.ca.gov
HIGHLIGHTS	Child-friendly, forest, history
LOWLIGHT	Low elevation

ROUTE | Walk toward the Donner Memorial and then head southwest behind some wooden buildings. Eventually, you draw near to Donner Creek and continue to a wooden bridge across the creek. At the far side of the bridge, follow the course of one of the campground roads generally south toward the east side of a pond. Loop around the pond along the base of Schallenberger Ridge to the vicinity of the Campfire Center and then head northeast back to the Donner Memorial.

C ▪ Coldstream Trail

LEVEL	Novice
LENGTH	2.1 miles, loop
TIME	Half day
ELEVATION	+250'–250'
DIFFICULTY	Easy
AVALANCHE RISK	Low
DOGS	Not allowed
FACILITIES	Museum, picnic areas, ranger station, restrooms
MAP	*Donner Memorial State Park Winter Trail Map* (web map)
MANAGEMENT	California State Parks at 530-582-7892, www.parks.ca.gov
HIGHLIGHTS	Child-friendly, history, stream
LOWLIGHT	Low elevation

ROUTE | [1] Walk toward the Donner Memorial and then head southwest behind some wooden buildings. Eventually, you draw near to Donner Creek and continue to a wooden bridge across the creek. At the far side of the bridge, follow the course of one of the campground roads generally south toward the east side of a pond. Beyond the pond, you intersect Coldstream Road [2] and follow it through Coldstream Valley for about one and three-quarters of a mile to the far (south) side of Merrill's Ponds. Loop around the pond and head back toward the trailhead between the ponds and Cold Creek. Where you meet your original tracks from the Donner Memorial, retrace your steps back to the museum.

MILESTONES
1: Start at trailhead; 2: Intersect Coldstream Road; 1: Return to trailhead.
[1] Walk toward the Donner Memorial

D ▪ Schallenberger Ridge Loop

Modern-day recreationists, armed with good equipment, reliable weather forecasts, and accurate maps, flock to an area that involved the Donner Party, perhaps the best-known tragedy of westward expansion. Over a century and a half later, outdoor adventurers can experience the beauty of a winter wonderland that was no doubt lost on these unfortunate pioneers. Donner Lake is beautiful in its own right, but travelers along Schallenberger Ridge enjoy the added bonus of stunning views of some of the Tahoe Sierra's most notable

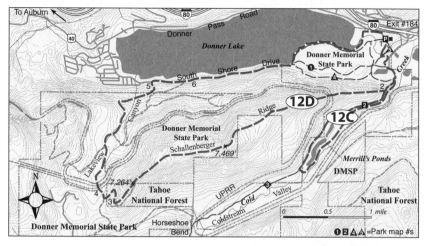

12C, D. Coldstream Trail and Schallenberger Ridge Loop

landmarks. Numerous peaks are visible, including Mount Lincoln, Anderson Peak, and Castle Peak. While visitors experience the bustle of activity in nearby Truckee and the whizzing of traffic along the concrete ribbon of Interstate 80, snowshoers and skiers may feel as though they are in a different world altogether while traveling along this remote crest route.

This trip, vaguely reminiscent of the grisly tale of the Donner Party, is not for everyone, as completing the full journey requires a good portion of the day, particularly when breaking trail in fresh powder is necessary. Although the route is generally straightforward, some route finding is necessary, especially when navigating a route down Lakeview Canyon. A potential drawback to the trip is the mile-long walk along the plowed section of road through the housing area on the south side of Donner Lake between Lakeview Canyon and the park.

LEVEL	Advanced
LENGTH	10 miles, loop
TIME	Full day
ELEVATION	+1,800'–1,800'
DIFFICULTY	Strenuous
AVALANCHE RISK	Moderate
DOGS	Not allowed
FACILITIES	Museum, picnic areas, ranger station, restrooms
MAP	*Donner Memorial State Park Winter Trail Map* (web map)
MANAGEMENT	California State Parks at 530-582-7892, www.parks.ca.gov
HIGHLIGHTS	Forest, history, lake, solitude, views
LOWLIGHTS	Mile-long walk on S. Shore Drive, railroad tracks crossing

TIP | Avoid the north edge of Schallenberger Ridge, where nasty cornices oftentimes are present.

ROUTE | [1] From the trailhead, follow the Coldstream Trail #2 to meet the nose of the east end of Schallenberger Ridge [2], about a mile from the parking area. Leave the road and climb moderately steeply up the nose of the ridge through a light forest of firs and pines. After the initial ascent, the terrain eases a bit, with filtered views down into Coldstream Valley and up toward the ridge between Anderson Peak and Mount Lincoln. Along the way to the high point at 7,469 feet, you climb through alternating areas of open ridge and light forest. Once at the apex of Schallenberger Ridge, 3 miles from the trailhead, views expand to include Donner Peak and Mount Judah to the west, Boreal Ridge and Castle Peak to the northwest, Mount Rose and the Carson Range to the east, and a host of additional landmarks, including Donner Lake, Interstate 80, and Donner Pass Road.

Descend along the ridge through light-to-scattered forest to a saddle and then make a short, moderate climb up the hill three-quarters of a mile west of Peak 7469. From there, a nearly level stroll along the ridge leads to improved views where the forest thins again. Soon the ridge narrows and you make a brief descent to the next saddle, followed by a short climb to the top of Peak 7264.

From Peak 7264, follow the narrow crest of Schallenberger Ridge on a moderate descent toward the broad, forested saddle above Lakeview Canyon. At four and three-quarter miles you meet a road in the saddle [3]. Unless you arrive immediately after a storm, there most likely will be plenty of tracks here, as snowmobilers frequently use this road as a connection between Donner Lake and Coldstream Valley.

Turn north and follow the road on a winding descent for one-quarter mile. Where you approach the railroad tracks, the road bends west and parallels the tracks for a half mile before crossing over and continuing down Lakeview Canyon. Rather than follow the road, carefully head straight down across the tracks near Eder [4], an abandoned railroad stop as shown on the *Norden* topographic map. Once safely across the tracks, you must negotiate the steep bank on the downhill side.

Beyond the tracks, head north across gentle terrain to the west branch of a seasonal creek draining Lakeview Canyon. Locate the continuation of the road nearby and follow its winding course down the canyon to the plowed road [5] above the south shore of Donner Lake, 7 miles from the trailhead.

For the next mile, you are forced to abandon the snowshoes and simply walk along the road past the homes on the south side of the lake. Once you reach the end of the plowed section of road [6], put on the snowshoes again and proceed on a gently descending grade on the way back into Donner Memorial State Park near China Cove, 8.5 miles from the trailhead.

Proceed through park property for a short distance to a groomed turnaround. Veer north at this point and follow the north branch of the Snowshoe Adventure Trail #4 around China Cove and east along the south shore of the lake. Just past the lake, remaining on Trail #4, you cross a bridge over Donner Creek and soon conclude the journey back at the parking lot [1].

THE DONNER PARTY Surprised by early season snows in November, members of the ill-fated Donner Party holed up near Donner Lake and attempted to survive the harsh conditions of the winter of 1846–1847. Out of the eighty-seven who began the trip in Illinois, only forty-seven were eventually rescued and led to safety over Donner Pass and down to more hospitable climes in the valleys of California. The museum at Donner Memorial State Park is an excellent place to gain a fuller understanding of this tragedy.

MILESTONES

1: Start at trailhead; 2: Leave Coldstream Trail and climb west on Schallenberger Ridge; 3: Turn right and follow road down Lakeview Canyon; 4: Cross railroad tracks at Eder; 5: Turn right at South Shore Drive; 6: Junction of Snowshoe Adventure Trail #4; 1: Return to trailhead.

GO GREEN | Volunteers are essential in the California State Park system. Opportunities include docents, visitor center volunteers, public safety, operations, maintenance, administration, and natural and cultural resource protection. For more information, visit the state park website at www.parks.ca.gov/?page_id=886, call 916-653-9069, or email: volunteer.inparksprogram@parks.ca.gov.

WARM-UPS | As the Schallenberger loop is a rigorous undertaking, Donner Lake Kitchen would be a fine place to eat breakfast before the trip. Located at 13720 Donner Pass Road, the family-owned café serves breakfast and lunch from 7:00 AM to 2:00 PM seven days a week. The huevos rancheros topped with chorizo is the house specialty.

TRIP 13 | Brockway Summit to Peak 7766

A short but steep ascent leads to supreme views of Lake Tahoe and the surrounding mountains. In the summer, hikers follow the Tahoe Rim Trail for about a mile to a junction with a spur trail up to this wonderful vista. However, snowfall has a way of obliterating well-defined summer trails, forcing winter users to find their own way. Actually following the alignment of this section of the TRT in winter is a daunting task, so the description below forsakes the summer route and instead climbs directly up the hillside to the top of Peak 7766.

Although the climb begins in fairly dense timber, the route is simple—climb up the slope until you can't climb any higher. Nearing the top, the forest opens up, which ultimately allows for a nearly unobstructed vista from the summit. The view of Lake Tahoe and surrounding peaks is a truly fine reward for the relatively brief effort.

LEVEL	Intermediate
LENGTH	1.25 miles, out and back
TIME	Half day
ELEVATION	+700'–0'
DIFFICULTY	Moderate
AVALANCHE RISK	Low
DOGS	OK
FACILITIES	None
MAP	USGS *Martis Peak*
MANAGEMENT	Lake Tahoe Basin Management Unit at 530-543-2600, www.fs.usda.gov/ltbmu
HIGHLIGHT	Views
LOWLIGHT	Limited parking

TIP | The nearby route from Brockway Summit to the Martis Peak Lookout used to be a favorite trip for both Nordic skiers and snowshoers. Unfortunately, a snowmobile concession has been operating on that route for several years, making it a somewhat unattractive proposition for the human-powered

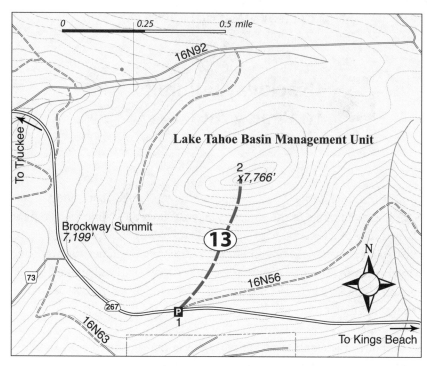

13. Brockway Summit to Peak 7766

crowd. Snowboarders and backcountry skiers should enjoy the short but fun ride down.

TRAILHEAD | 39°15.499'N, 120°03.898'W Drive Highway 267, either southbound from Truckee or northbound from Kings Beach, to the plowed shoulder just a half mile east of Brockway Summit. Depending on the depth of the snow, you may find hiker emblems or Tahoe Rim Trail signs alongside the highway.

ROUTE | [1] Cross Highway 267 to the northeast shoulder and head up snow-covered Forest Road 16N56 a short distance to the site of the summer trailhead. The TRT bends west from here, but discerning the route of the snow-covered trail is difficult beyond a series of switchbacks zigzagging up the moderately forested hillside. Instead, you climb moderately steeply directly toward the ridge crest above. Continue through dense Jeffrey pine forest, and, even though the trees prohibit you from gaining your bearings on the initial ascent, the route finding is simple—just head for the top. The higher you climb, the less dense the forest becomes, granting your eyes a small prelude to the upcoming vista from the top of the mountain. Once you reach the sparsely forested and long ridge leading to the summit [2], Lake Tahoe and the surrounding mountains are revealed in all their glory.

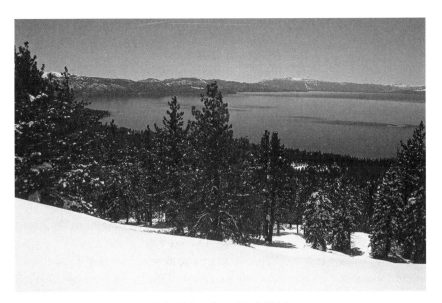

Lake Tahoe from Peak 7766

A clear day promises exquisite views of one of California's most prominent natural treasures. Lake Tahoe shimmers in the midwinter sun, surrounded by a ring of Sierra peaks. Some of the more noteworthy summits include Silver Peak above the Truckee River canyon to the west, Mount Tallac towering above the southwest shore and backdropped by the rugged peaks of Desolation Wilderness, the triangular summit of 10,881-foot Freel Peak rising above the southeast shore as Tahoe's highest mountain, and the eastside summit of Snow Valley Peak. Nearby is Martis Peak, where keen eyes may spy the lookout nestled on a ridgetop immediately northwest of the true summit.

TAHOE RIM TRAIL Hidden from sight by a blanket of snow in the winter, at one time in the not-so-distant past, the Tahoe Rim Trail didn't even exist in this area of the Lake Tahoe Basin Management Unit. Unlike sections of existing tread that were incorporated into the TRT, such as the Pacific Crest Trail, much of the tread in the north and east parts of the basin had to be constructed. Under the inspiration and supervision of Forest Ranger Glenn Hampton, who came to be known as the "Father of the Tahoe Rim Trail," numerous volunteers spent thousands of hours to complete the missing segments of the 165-mile loop trail. Officially dedicated in 2001, the TRT has become one of the premier long-distance trails in the American West.

Just beyond Martis Peak to the southeast is Mount Baldy, lying just inside the Mount Rose Wilderness. After thoroughly enjoying the view, retrace your steps to the trailhead [1].

MILESTONES

1: Start at trailhead; 2: Top of Peak 7766; 1: Return to trailhead.

GO GREEN | Although primarily a group dedicated to warm-weather pursuits, you can volunteer time or donate money to the Tahoe Rim Trail by visiting their website at tahoerimtrail.org.

OPTIONS | While there exists plenty of backcountry to explore beyond Peak 7766, be prepared for some challenging navigation.

WARM-UPS | Since its opening in 1981, the Log Cabin Café in Kings Beach (8692 North Lake Boulevard) has been voted more than once as the best place for breakfast in North Tahoe. The small café serves up ample portions of home cooking, with a number of unique dishes (the Cajun Eggs Benedict is a spicy twist on the traditional dish and was featured in *Bon Appétit* magazine). Open seven days a week from 7:00 AM to 2:00 PM, the popular restaurant can be quite busy on weekends. However, the café does allow you to call ahead to be placed on their waiting list (530-546-7109).

TRIP

14 | Tamarack Lake

Winter enthusiasts looking for a quick and relatively easy trip will find the journey to Tamarack Lake a good option, as the distance is short and the terrain fairly gentle except for a short, moderate stretch of climbing. Nestled beneath the shadow of Tamarack Peak, the lake and surrounding meadow are quite picturesque, with the combination of pleasant scenery and easy terrain providing a fine destination for a quick trip to the mountains.

LEVEL	Novice
LENGTH	1 mile, out and back
TIME	2 hours
ELEVATION	+200'–0'
DIFFICULTY	Easy
AVALANCHE RISK	Low
DOGS	OK
FACILITIES	None
MAPS	USGS *Mount Rose*; USFS *Mount Rose Wilderness*
MANAGEMENT	USFS Humboldt-Toiyabe National Forest, Carson Ranger District at 775-882-2766, www.fs.usda.gov/htnf
HIGHLIGHT	Lake
LOWLIGHT	Highway crossing

TIPS: Keep an eye out for backcountry skiers and boarders, as Tamarack Peak is a favorite of the downhill crowd. This trip is best done in the morning or midday, as the lake basin is shaded by Tamarack Peak in the afternoon.

TRAILHEAD | 39°19.283'N, 119°54.157'W Follow the Mount Rose Highway (NV State Route 431) to a cleared shoulder 1 mile northbound of the Mount Rose Highway Summit.

ROUTE | [1] From the parking area, carefully cross the highway to the west side and scale the snowbank. Head southwest away from the highway to the east side of a tributary of Galena Creek draining Tamarack Lake. Make a brief ascent of a forested hillside to the apex of a gently sloping ridge and follow it to the east shore of snow-covered Tamarack Lake [2]. From there you can

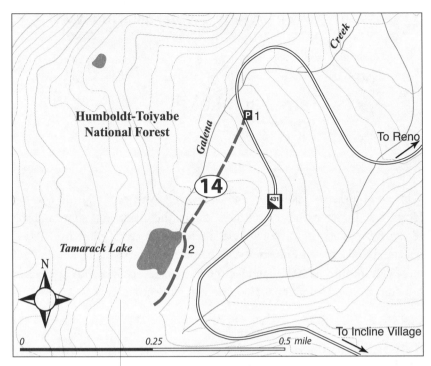

14. Tamarack Lake

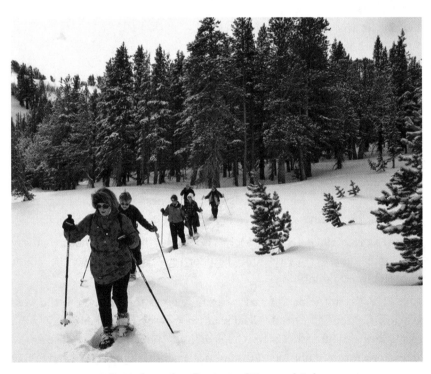

Snowshoers heading toward Tamarack Lake

TAMARACK (*Larix occidentalis*) The tamarack tree refers to a member of the larch family and is not found in the Sierra Nevada. The tamarack does grow in the mountains of the Pacific Northwest, northern Rockies, and Canada. The trees were most likely confused with lodgepole pines (*Pinus contorta*), which are common in the Mount Rose area. A unique feature of the tamarack is that they are deciduous conifers. Unlike other "evergreens," the tamarack's needles turn a beautiful golden color in autumn and then fall to the ground like the leaves of other deciduous trees. In the spring, tamarack can be easily identified by their brand new, bright green needles.

continue across the lake and open meadow to the south before retracing your steps to the parking area [1].

MILESTONES

1: Start at parking area; 2: Tamarack Lake; 1: Return to parking area.

GO GREEN | Friends of Nevada Wilderness have been quite active within the Mount Rose Wilderness. Check out their website at www.nevadawilderness .org.

OPTIONS | With extra time and energy, you could continue up steeper terrain toward Tamarack Peak (see Map 16 Galena Creek–Third Creek Loop).

WARM-UPS | Since the unfortunate closing of the Christmas Tree restaurant, you'll have to go all the way down to Reno to find a decent café or watering hole. The Sunrise Café just off the Mount Rose Highway (18603 Wedge Parkway) would be a fine stop for one of their fresh breakfast dishes on the way to the trailhead. Open seven days a week from 7:00 AM to 2:00 PM, you can check out their menu at www.sunrisecafereno.com.

TRIP

15 | Fireplug

LEVEL	Intermediate
LENGTH	1 mile, out and back
TIME	Half day
ELEVATION	+600'–0'
DIFFICULTY	Moderate
AVALANCHE RISK	Moderate
DOGS	OK
FACILITIES	None
MAPS	USGS *Mount Rose*; USFS *Mount Rose Wilderness*
MANAGEMENT	USFS Humboldt-Toiyabe National Forest, Carson Ranger District at 775-882-2766, www.fs.usda.gov/htnf

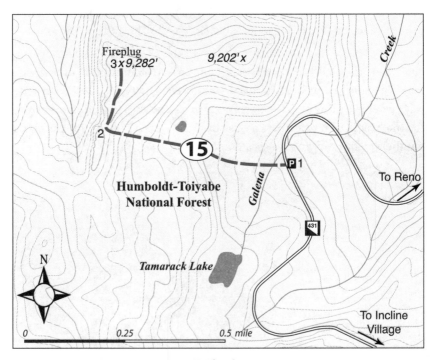

15. Fireplug

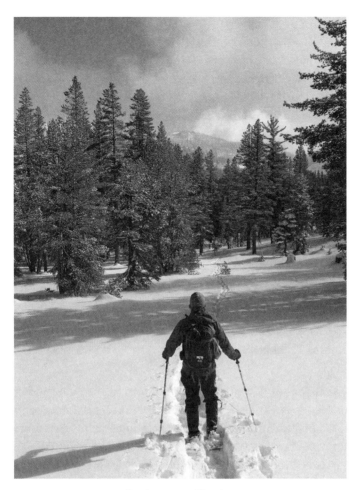

On the way to Fireplug

HIGHLIGHT Views

LOWLIGHT Steep

TIP | Keep an eye out for backcountry skiers and boarders, as Tamarack Peak is a favorite of the downhill crowd.

TRAILHEAD | 39°19.283'N, 119°54.157'W Follow the Mount Rose Highway (NV State Route 431) to a cleared shoulder 1 mile north of Mount Rose Summit.

ROUTE | [1] From the parking area, carefully cross the highway to the west side and scale the snowbank. Follow a moderately ascending route through light forest for about one-quarter mile to where the grade steepens considerably. Head steeply toward a saddle [2] in the ridge above and then turn generally north along the ridge to gain the top [3] and a beautiful view of the surrounding countryside. When the time comes, retrace your steps to the trailhead [1].

LODGEPOLE PINE (*Pinus contorta*) Mistakenly called tamarack pine, lodgepole pine is one of the most widely distributed pines in the American West. Easily identified as the only pine with two-needle bundles in the region, the tree is typically found in areas of sufficient groundwater, such as near lakes and streams, or on the edge of meadows and bogs. Often present in pure stands, in the Tahoe area they can also be found in a mixed forest with mountain hemlocks, western white pines, and red firs, or with whitebark pines in the higher elevations.

MILESTONES

1: Start at trailhead; 2: Saddle; 3: Top of Fireplug; 1: Return to trailhead.

GO GREEN | Great Basin Institute is a research- and education-based organization in Nevada offering a variety of programs. Check out their website at www.thegreatbasininstitute.org.

OPTIONS | With extra time and energy, continuing beyond the lake up steeper terrain toward Tamarack Peak is possible (see Map 16 Galena Creek–Third Creek Loop).

WARM-UPS | In Incline Village near the terminus of the famous Flume Trail mountain bike route, Tunnel Creek Café serves breakfast items, sandwiches, and soups, along with coffee drinks and premium beers. Open seven days a week from 8:00 AM to 4:00 PM, you can find the café just off State Route 28 at 1115 Tunnel Creek Road. See their menu at www.tunnelcreekcafe.com.

TRIP 16

Galena Creek–Third Creek Loop

LEVEL	Intermediate
LENGTH	5.8 miles, loop
TIME	Three-quarter day
ELEVATION	+850'–850'
DIFFICULTY	Moderate to strenuous
AVALANCHE RISK	Low to moderate
DOGS	OK
FACILITIES	None
MAPS	USGS *Mount Rose*; USFS *Mount Rose Wilderness*
MANAGEMENT	Humboldt-Toiyabe National Forest, Carson Ranger District at 775-882-2766, www.fs.usda.gov/htnf; Lake Tahoe Basin Management Unit at 530-543-2600, www.fs.usda.gov/ltbmu
HIGHLIGHTS	Scenery, views
LOWLIGHT	Snowmobiles (1 mile of route)

TIP | As the Relay Ridge Road is also a popular ski route, remember to stay out of any fresh ski tracks.

TRAILHEAD | 39°18.792'N, 119°53.843'W Follow the Mount Rose Highway (NV State Route 431) to Mount Rose Summit, which at 8,900 feet is the highest year-round pass in the Sierra. Park your vehicle in the plowed area on the west side of the highway, which serves as the summer trailhead for the Mount Rose and Tahoe Rim Trails.

ROUTE | [1] From the parking area, ascend a short but steep slope and then follow a rising traverse along the ridge above the highway across mostly open slopes dotted with lodgepole and whitebark pines. Fine views of Tahoe Meadows and Lake Tahoe are plentiful from the ridgetop before the route veers away from the highway on the way to a saddle [2] between Peak 9201 on the right and Tamarack Peak on the left.

From the saddle, follow a slightly rising traverse across the eastern flank of Tamarack Peak, as mountain hemlocks join the pines. Mount Rose can be

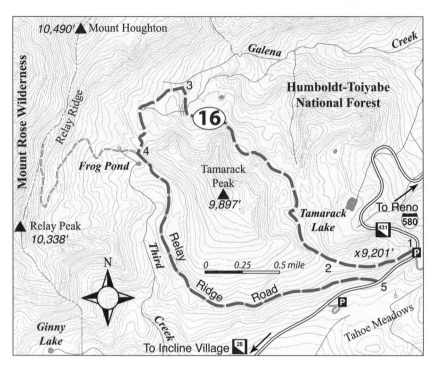

16. Galena Creek–Third Creek Loop

seen over the tops of the trees at various points along this traverse. About 1.5 miles from the parking lot, you begin a mild descent across steep slopes on the northeast side of Tamarack Peak toward the floor of Galena Creek. At the bottom of the descent, the route veers north across the basin and climbs moderately along the fringe of a large meadow to the north tributary of Galena Creek [3].

On the far side of the creek, turn southwest and follow the course of a jeep road paralleling a set of utility poles steeply upslope. A more moderate ascent arcs around the head of the canyon toward a saddle and the snow-covered Relay Ridge Road (FS 17N85) just beyond [4]. For the next mile of the route, you may encounter snowmobiles traveling the terrain west of the road.

Turn left (southeast) and follow the service road on a moderate descent across the forested slopes above Third Creek. As you progress and the road bends around the south flank of Tamarack Peak, the trees begin to thin, allowing fine views to the southwest of Lake Tahoe and the distant peaks in Desolation Wilderness above the southwest shore. Below lies the open plain of Tahoe Meadows backdropped by Slide Mountain. Eventually the road meets the Mount Rose Highway [5] near a concrete block building. The Mount Rose trailhead parking lot is 0.3 mile up the highway—you can either walk up the

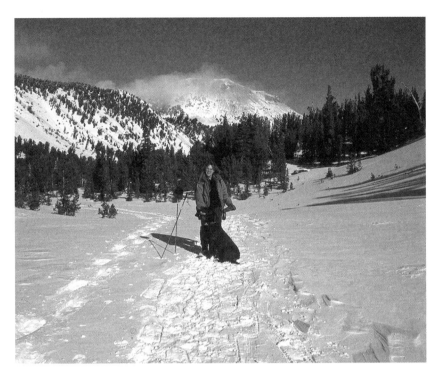
Along upper Galena Creek

shoulder or make an ascending traverse across the slope above to get back to your vehicle [1].

MILESTONES

1: Start at Mount Rose trailhead; 2: Saddle; 3: Turn left at jeep road; 4: Turn left at Relay Ridge Road; 5: Mount Rose Highway; 1: Return to trailhead.

GO GREEN | You can assist the Humboldt-Toiyabe National Forest by volunteering for short-term or seasonal projects. For more information, visit the volunteer page at www.fs.usda.gov/main/r4/jobs/volunteer.

GALENA CREEK RESORT? Way back in the 1980s, the area in the upper Galena Creek drainage was in peril of being developed into a destination resort complete with casino, condominiums, golf course, and ski area. The tranquil meadows and groves of lodgepole pines would have been sacrificed for such commercialism. Fortunately, a contingent of Nevada lawmakers worked out a land exchange with the developers, swapping the Galena Creek property for lands in southern Nevada.

OPTIONS | If you wish to avoid the possibility of encountering snowmobiles altogether, climbing up the north ridge of Tamarack Peak to the summit and then descending the south slope to the Relay Ridge Road is possible.

WARM-UPS | Bagel lovers will find plenty of options to satisfy their passion at the Truckee Bagel Company in south Reno just off the Mount Rose Highway (18130 Wedge Parkway in the Raley's Shopping Center). A fine stop for either breakfast or lunch on the way to or from the trailhead, you can check out their menus at www.truckeebagelcompany.com.

TRIP

17 Tamarack Peak

LEVEL	Intermediate
LENGTH	3.2 miles, out and back
TIME	Half day
ELEVATION	+950'–0'
DIFFICULTY	Moderate to strenuous
AVALANCHE RISK	Moderate
DOGS	OK
FACILITIES	None
MAPS	USGS *Mount Rose*; USFS *Mount Rose Wilderness*
MANAGEMENT	Humboldt-Toiyabe National Forest, Carson Ranger District at 775-882-2766, www.fs.usda.gov/htnf; Lake Tahoe Basin Management Unit at 530-543-2600, www.fs.usda.gov/ltbmu
HIGHLIGHTS	Scenery, summit, views
LOWLIGHT	Snowmobiles (1 mile of route)

TIP | Avoid this trip during periods of strong winds.

TRAILHEAD | 39°18.792'N, 119°53.843'W Follow the Mount Rose Highway (NV State Route 431) to Mount Rose Summit, which at 8,900 feet is the highest year-round pass in the Sierra. Park your vehicle in the plowed area on the west side of the highway, which serves as the summer trailhead for the Mount Rose and Tahoe Rim Trails.

ROUTE | [1] From the parking area, ascend a short but steep slope and then follow a rising traverse along the ridge above the highway across mostly open slopes dotted with lodgepole and whitebark pines. Fine views of Tahoe Meadows and Lake Tahoe are plentiful from the ridge top before the route veers away from the highway on the way to a saddle [2] between Peak 9201 on the right and Tamarack Peak on the left.

From the saddle, ascend the southeast ridge of Tamarack Peak on a stiff climb through the trees. Soon the forest starts to thin, where you are afforded find views of Lake Tahoe and the surrounding terrain. Continue up the ridge,

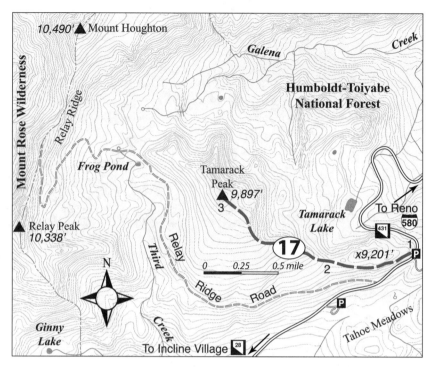

17. Tamarack Peak

steeply at times, eventually topping out at the 9,897-foot summit of Tamarack Peak [3]. After thoroughly enjoying the magnificent view, retrace your steps to the trailhead [1].

MILESTONES

1: Start at Mount Rose trailhead; 2: Saddle; 3: Summit of Tamarack Peak; 1: Return to trailhead.

GO GREEN | You can support conservation of the north Tahoe region by joining the Sierra Club, either through the Toiyabe (sierraclub.org/toiyabe) or Mother Lode (sierraclub.org/mother-lode) Chapters.

TAMARACK (*Larix occidentalis*) Similar to Tamarack Lake, Tamarack Peak was named for the tamarack tree. The true tamarack is a member of the larch family and is not found in the Sierra Nevada. The tamarack does grow in the mountains of the Pacific Northwest, northern Rockies, and Canada. The trees were most likely confused with lodgepole pines (*Pinus contorta*), which are common in the Mount Rose area.

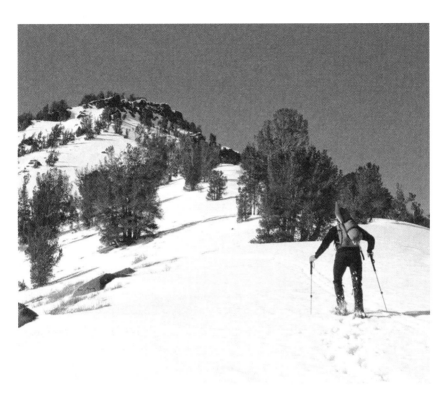

On the ridge to Tamarack Peak

OPTIONS | To extend the trip, continue down the northwest ridge to either the Relay Ridge Road or the route of the old Mount Rose Trail and then loop back to the trailhead.

WARM-UPS | The Wildflower Café in Incline Village (869 Tahoe Boulevard) has been feeding locals and tourists fine food for breakfast and lunch for over thirty years. You can see their menus at www.wildflowercafetahoe.com.

18 | Mount Rose

Hundreds of hikers may reach the summit of Mount Rose on a busy summer weekend, but only a few daring souls accept the challenge of an ascent during the winter months. Views from the third-highest peak in the Tahoe Basin are sublime, a more than worthwhile reward for the extreme effort involved. Most winter enthusiasts are content with snowshoeing shorter routes nearby, but the challenge of ascending Mount Rose appeals to more experienced snowshoers. The first half of the trip follows the summer route of the single-track Mount Rose Trail on a mellow traverse around the east and north slopes of Tamarack Peak before descending into the upper Galena Creek drainage. From there, the going gets tough, requiring steep ascents and often less than ideal snow conditions on the upper mountain. For those who prevail, the scenery is spectacular.

LEVEL	Extreme
LENGTH	10 miles, out and back
TIME	Full day
ELEVATION	+2,100'–325'
DIFFICULTY	Very strenuous
AVALANCHE RISK	Moderate to high
DOGS	OK
FACILITIES	None
MAPS	USGS *Mount Rose*; USFS *Mount Rose Wilderness*
MANAGEMENT	Humboldt-Toiyabe National Forest, Carson Ranger District at 775-882-2766, www.fs.usda.gov/htnf
HIGHLIGHTS	Scenery, summit, views
LOWLIGHTS	Steep, wind-prone

TIP | This can be an extreme undertaking requiring stamina and good navigational skills. Frigid temperatures with strong winds are possible, with conditions varying greatly between the trailhead and the summit. Everyone in your group should be experienced and properly equipped. Get an early start to finish the trip before dark.

TRAILHEAD | 39°18.792'N, 119°53.843'W Follow the Mount Rose Highway (NV State Route 431) to Mount Rose Summit, which at 8,900 feet is the highest year-round pass in the Sierra. Park your vehicle in the plowed area on the west side of the highway, which serves as the summer trailhead for the Mount Rose and Tahoe Rim Trails.

ROUTE | [1] From the parking area, ascend a short but steep slope and then follow a rising traverse along the ridge above the highway across mostly open slopes dotted with lodgepole and whitebark pines. Fine views of Tahoe Meadows and Lake Tahoe are plentiful from the ridgetop before the route

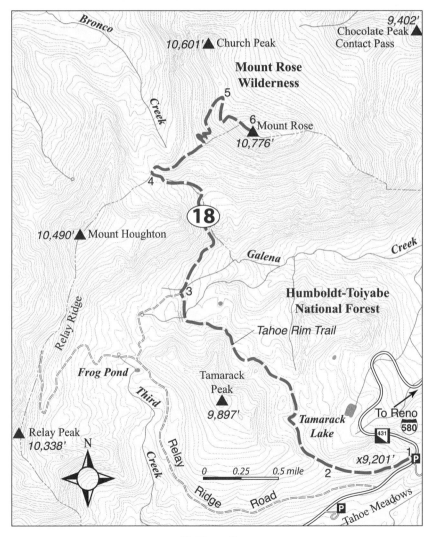

18. Mount Rose

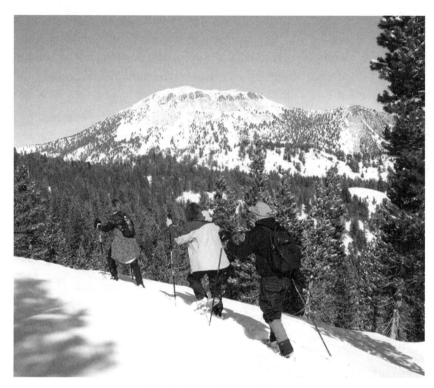
Headed toward Mount Rose

veers away from the highway on the way to a saddle [2] between Peak 9201 on the right and Tamarack Peak on the left.

From the saddle, follow a slightly rising traverse across the eastern flank of Tamarack Peak, as mountain hemlocks join the pines. Mount Rose can be seen over the tops of the trees at various points along this traverse. About 1.5 miles from the parking lot, you begin a mild descent across steep slopes on the northeast side of Tamarack Peak toward the floor of Galena Creek. At the bottom of the descent, the route veers north across the basin and climbs moderately along the fringe of a large meadow to the north tributary of Galena Creek [3].

Cross the creek and make a moderate ascent across an open hillside to a side canyon, where you turn northwest up a much steeper grade. Technically, this will be the most difficult stretch, as the angle of the slope is severe and an unfortunate slip would send you careening toward the bottom of the canyon. Complicating matters, the snow may be wind packed through here as well. Crest a ridge at the head of the canyon [4], where you enter the Mount Rose Wilderness. Turn right and head northeast along the ridge. If the winds are howling, this would be a good place to turn around and head back, as they will only become worse near the summit. Continue on the ridge for a half mile until you encounter the summit massif of Mount Rose, where the route climbs northwest up the slope. After gaining another 200 feet of elevation, make an ascending traverse toward the broad saddle [5] between Mount Rose and 10,601-foot-high Church Peak. More than likely the snow will be wind packed here as well, so watch your footing. At the saddle, turn southeast and ascend steeply up the final slopes to the top [6].

The views from the summit of Mount Rose are quite impressive. On clear days following storms, the northward views may extend all the way past Lassen Peak to Mount Shasta. If the atmosphere is hazier, Sierra Buttes will be the prominent landmark in that direction. Above the southwest shore of Lake Tahoe, the dark hulk of Mount Tallac and the symmetrical summit of Pyramid Peak stand guard over Desolation Wilderness. To the south, the tri-peaks of Freel Peak, Jobs Peak, and Jobs Sister are the dominant summits of the Carson Range. As expected, the crystalline waters of Lake Tahoe provide the centerpiece for the grandest of summit views.

If the winds on top of Mount Rose are calm, consider yourself fortunate. If not, your continued admiration of the views will probably be short-lived, as you will most likely be anxious to return to the less breezy conditions lower on the mountain. However long your stay, the short daylight hours of winter will ultimately hasten your return, as you retrace your steps to the trailhead [1].

WHITEBARK PINE (*Pinus albicaulis*) This member of the pine family with bundles of five needles is found in the high, subalpine elevations of the Carson Range. On exposed ridgetops, trees may be dwarfed and multitrunked, sometimes forming shrubby mats called *krummholz*. When present, distinctive purplish cones easily identify the tree, but the cones that aren't destroyed by Clark's Nutcrackers in their pursuit of whitebark pine seeds tend to crumble on the branches and become buried by winter snows.

MILESTONES

1: Start at Mount Rose trailhead; 2: Saddle; 3: Galena Creek crossing; 4: Turn right at ridge crest; 5: Saddle between Mount Rose and Church Peak; 6: Summit of Mount Rose; 1: Return to trailhead.

GO GREEN | Snowlands Network is a fine organization dedicated to protecting winter human-powered recreation across public lands. Consult their website at www.snowlands.org.

OPTIONS | More than likely, a successful ascent of Mount Rose will be enough of an effort for the strongest of outdoor enthusiasts. The extremely hardy could double-summit by ascending Church Peak from the saddle on the way down from the summit of Rose.

WARM-UPS | In Incline Village near the terminus of the famous Flume Trail mountain bike route, Tunnel Creek Café serves breakfast items, sandwiches, and soups, along with coffee drinks and premium beers. Open seven days a week from 8:00 AM to 4:00 PM, you can find the café just off State Route 28 at 1115 Tunnel Creek Road. See their menu at www.tunnelcreekcafe.com.

TRIP
19 Relay Peak

A moderate climb along the broad course of the Relay Ridge Road leads to the bottom of Relay Ridge, where the road adopts a stiffer course on the way to the crest. From there, a half-mile climb along the north ridge leads to the summit, where magnificent views unfold in every direction.

LEVEL	Advanced to extreme
LENGTH	9.6 miles, out and back
TIME	Full day
ELEVATION	+1,400'–0'
DIFFICULTY	Strenuous
AVALANCHE RISK	Moderate to high
DOGS	OK
FACILITIES	None
MAPS	USGS *Mount Rose*; USFS *Mount Rose Wilderness*
MANAGEMENT	Humboldt-Toiyabe National Forest, Carson Ranger District at 775-882-2766, www.fs.usda.gov/htnf; Lake Tahoe Basin Management Unit at 530-543-2600, www.fs.usda.gov/ltbmu
HIGHLIGHTS	Summit, views
LOWLIGHT	Snowmobiles

TIP | This can be an extreme undertaking requiring stamina and good navigational skills. Frigid temperatures with strong winds are possible, with conditions varying greatly between the trailhead and the summit. Everyone in your group should be experienced and properly equipped. Get an early start to finish the trip before dark.

TRAILHEAD | 39°18.611'N, 119°54.087'W Follow the Mount Rose Highway (NV State Route 431) to a concrete block building above the north shoulder of the highway, 0.3 mile southwest of Mount Rose Summit. Park your vehicle along the shoulder as space allows.

ROUTE | [1] Leave the highway and follow the snow-covered surface of well-graded Forest Service Road 17N85. Scattered lodgepole pines alternately

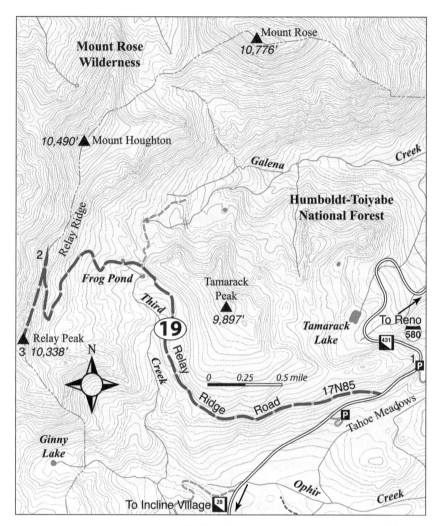

19. Relay Peak

block and allow increasingly spectacular views to the southwest of shimmering Lake Tahoe and the snowy peaks of Desolation Wilderness above the far shore. Below is the broad expanse of Tahoe Meadows, one of the region's favorite winter playgrounds. The road eventually bends around to the northwest below Tamarack Peak, where the chance of encountering snowmobiles becomes a possibility. Leaving the lake views behind, you continue the steady ascent through denser forest cover. Follow the road on an arcing ascent around the head of the canyon of Third Creek.

The road begins a series of three switchbacks that lead stiffly up the east face of Relay Ridge (of course, you could take a more direct approach if you want to climb even more steeply). After the long zigzagging ascent, you crest

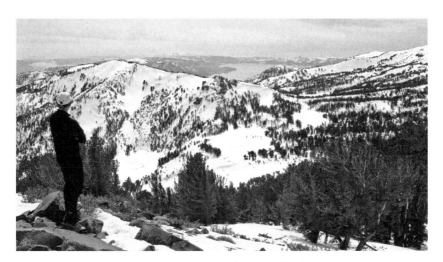
Lake Tahoe view from the shoulder of Relay Peak

Relay Ridge [2], obviously named for the preponderance of communication equipment carpeting the ridge.

Head south-southwest along the ridge past the man-made structures and towers and continue toward the top of Relay Peak. A moderate, half-mile climb leads to the 10,338-foot summit [3], where a marvelous view unfolds of most of the Lake Tahoe Basin. Below and to the southeast is Tahoe Meadows and a slice of Washoe Lake beyond appearing through the gash of Ophir Creek Canyon and backdropped by rows of desert ranges parading into the Great Basin. The Carson Range summits of Mount Houghton and Mount Rose dominate the immediate area to the northeast. On clear days, to the distant north you may be able to see all the way to Lassen Peak and Mount Shasta. Closer in that direction are the spires of Sierra Buttes. Many other notable Tahoe Sierra landmarks are visible, too numerous to mention—packing along a small-scale map of the area will allow you to identify them. When your time is finished, retrace your steps to the trailhead [1].

RELAY PEAK This 10,335-foot summit is so named for the preponderance of radio towers lining adjacent Relay Ridge. The road to the ridge was constructed for maintenance purposes. Careful observation may note some old structures near the service road at the base of the ridge, where a tram used to transport materials up the steep slope to the top of the ridge. The road is a popular mountain bike route in the summer. Relay Peak holds the distinction of being the highest point along the Tahoe Rim Trail.

1: Start at trailhead; 2: Relay Ridge; 3: Summit of Relay Peak; 1: Return to trailhead.

GO GREEN | Friends of Nevada Wilderness have been quite active within the Mount Rose Wilderness. Check out their website at www.nevadawilderness .org.

OPTIONS | More than likely, a successful ascent of Relay Peak will be enough of an effort for the strongest of outdoor recreationists. Those with extra energy could double-summit by climbing Mount Houghton.

WARM-UPS | Since the unfortunate closing of the Christmas Tree restaurant, you'll have to go all the way down to Reno to find a decent café or watering hole. Sunrise Café just off the Mount Rose Highway (18603 Wedge Parkway) would be a fine stop for one of their fresh breakfast dishes on the way to the trailhead. Open seven days a week from 7:00 AM to 2:00 PM, you can check out their menu at www.sunrisecafereno.com.

20 Tahoe Meadows

Tahoe Meadows is a very popular winter playground for residents of Reno-Sparks and North Tahoe, where a weekend of clear skies and fresh powder attracts hundreds of winter enthusiasts to the wide-open terrain and gentle slopes. The Forest Service wisely banned the use of snowmobiles on the southeast side of the highway many years ago, restricting their presence to the northwest side, away from the heavily used meadows. While the area is covered with snowshoers, Nordic skiers, and families involved in snow play on weekends, a high percentage of the crowd seems reluctant to venture too far away from the highway. Snowshoers and skiers can often leave the masses behind by venturing into the trees surrounding the meadow, or by traveling down Ophir Creek toward Price Lake (see Options).

LEVEL	Novice to intermediate
LENGTH	Varies, loop or out and back hours to half day
TIME	House to half day
ELEVATION	Varies, +300'–300' maximum
DIFFICULTY	Easy
AVALANCHE RISK	Low
DOGS	OK
FACILITIES	Vault toilets
MAPS	USGS *Mount Rose*; USFS *Mount Rose Wilderness*
MANAGEMENT	Humboldt-Toiyabe National Forest, Carson Ranger District at 775-882-2766, www.fs.usda.gov/htnf; Lake Tahoe Basin Management Unit at 530-543-2600, www.fs.usda.gov/ltbmu
HIGHLIGHTS	Meadow, scenery
LOWLIGHT	Popular

TIP | The crowds seem to diminish a bit on weekdays.

TRAILHEAD | 39°18.485'N, 119°54.455'W Follow the Mount Rose Highway (Nevada State Route 431) to the Tahoe Rim Trail parking area, 0.7 mile southwest of Mount Rose Summit.

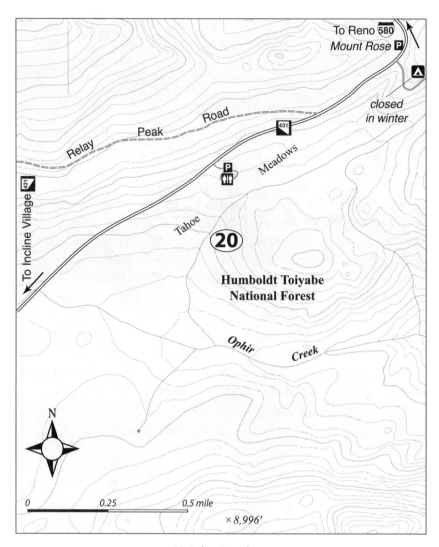

20. Tahoe Meadows

ROUTE | The great thing about Tahoe Meadows is the ability to tailor your trip to the skill level of your group and the time they have available. Loops around the meadows of varying lengths are quite easy to organize to fit any group's agenda. Chilling winds do blow across the open meadows at times, when heading for the shelter of the trees along the edge would be a wise alternative.

GO GREEN | You can support conservation of the north Tahoe region by joining the Sierra Club, either through the Toiyabe (sierraclub.org/toiyabe) or Mother Lode (sierraclub.org/mother-lode) Chapters.

OPTIONS | A fine alternative for a longer trip would be to head east across the meadows and down into Ophir Creek canyon. The grade starts out fairly

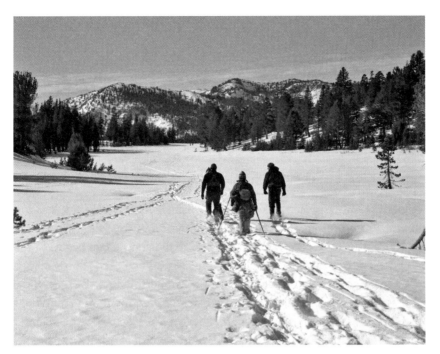
Snowshoers in Tahoe Meadows

gentle but gets steeper the farther you travel downstream. Continuing all the way to Price Lake is feasible, provided you save enough time and energy for the 2.5 mile uphill climb back to the car.

WARM-UPS | Bagel lovers will find plenty of options to satisfy their passion at the Truckee Bagel Company in south Reno just off the Mount Rose Highway (18130 Wedge Parkway in the Raley's Shopping Center). A fine stop for either breakfast or lunch on the way to or from the trailhead, you can check out their menus at www.truckeebagelcompany.com.

SLIDE MOUNTAIN   Just east of Tahoe Meadows stands aptly named Slide Mountain. Mark Twain wrote about the peak's recurrent habit of periodically sloughing away part of its real estate in his tale of the West, *Roughing It*. The most recent event occurred on Memorial Day weekend of 1983, when a landslide of moisture-saturated soils fell into Lower Price Lake, triggering a muddy torrent of sludge that roared down the canyon of Ophir Creek and spilled across Washoe Valley, blocking the freeway for several days. In the process, seven homes were destroyed and one person lost his life. The question is not if Slide Mountain will slide again but when.

Chickadee Ridge
and Peak 9225

Tahoe Meadows is a busy place in winter, especially on weekends. You can minimize the presence of your fellow humans a bit by following a short section of the Tahoe Rim Trail to Chickadee Ridge. The trip begins in the meadows, passes through a lodgepole pine forest, and then shortly climbs up to the apex of the Carson Range for a wonderful view of Lake Tahoe. The ridge received its name from the black-headed mountain chickadees frequently seen in the area. Most groups seem to be satisfied with the initial viewpoint along the ridge as their turnaround point, but farther wanderings are quite possible.

LEVEL	Novice to intermediate
LENGTH	3 miles, out and back
TIME	Half day
ELEVATION	+650'–0'
DIFFICULTY	Moderate
AVALANCHE RISK	Low to moderate
DOGS	OK
FACILITIES	None
MAPS	USGS *Mount Rose*; USFS *Mount Rose Wilderness*
MANAGEMENT	Humboldt-Toiyabe National Forest, Carson Ranger District at 775-882-2766, www.fs.usda.gov/htnf; Lake Tahoe Basin Management Unit at 530-543-2600, www.fs.usda.gov/ltbmu
HIGHLIGHTS	Meadow, scenery, views
LOWLIGHTS	Popular

TIP | A majority of visitors seem content with the first view of Tahoe from Chickadee Ridge as their turnaround point.

TRAILHEAD | 39°18.284'N, 119°54.890'W Follow the Mount Rose Highway (Nevada State Route 431) to the southwest edge of Tahoe Meadows and park along the shoulder as space allows.

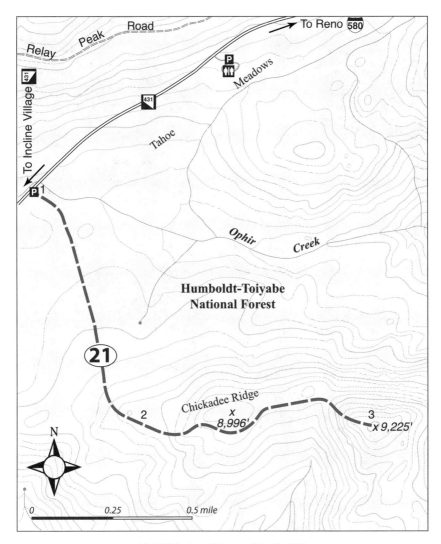

21. Chickadee Ridge and Peak 9225

ROUTE | [1] From the southwest edge of the meadows, head south on a gentle grade into lodgepole pine forest. Soon you begin climbing, gently at first and then more moderately on the approach to the base of the hill below Chickadee Ridge. Small meadows and occasional gaps in the forest may help you gain your bearings for the upcoming ascent. Climb more stiffly up the nose of the ridge through scattered whitebark pines on the way toward the top, where Lake Tahoe suddenly springs into view in all its glory. Traverse across the hillside on the west side of the ridge with nearly continuous lake views as your companion. By gaining the crest of Chickadee Ridge [2], the views expand to include Tahoe Meadows below and Mount Rose across the highway.

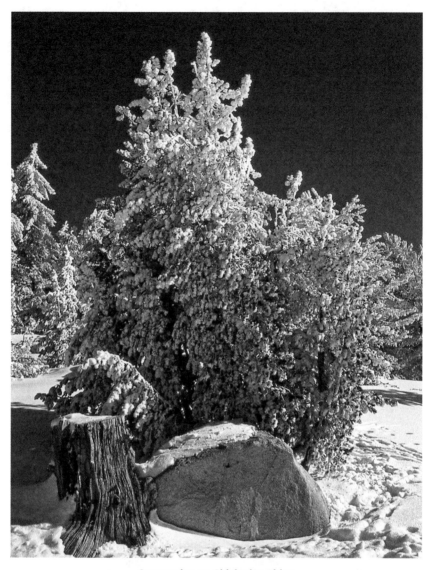

Snowy pine on Chickadee Ridge

Once on top of Chickadee Ridge, you can extend the trip as far as you desire. A nearby goal for intermediate snowshoers is the top of Peak 9225. To get there, follow the ridge to the base of the peak. The final climb to the top will prove to be too steep for skis, but experienced snowshoers can negotiate the final 200 feet with some difficulty. Depending on snow conditions, you may have to skirt some exposed boulders on the way and the snow may be wind packed, but the even grander view from the summit of Peak 9225 [3] is a worthy reward for all the sweat equity: Lake Tahoe lies at your feet, the peaks of Desolation Wilderness appear above the far shore, and Tahoe

MOUNTAIN CHICKADEE (*Parus gambeli*) This delightful little songbird of the mountain West is commonly seen and heard in this section of the Carson Range, frequently uttering their *chick-a-dee* call to anyone who listens. They are quite acrobatic, clinging to the underside of branches to pluck insects or seeds from cones with their short bills. A common practice on Chickadee Ridge is to place a small pile of birdseed in your palm and wait for the birds to eat from your hand, which they seem to be more than willing to do, especially in winter when food is more scarce. This practice is not recommended by some wildlife officials—if you plan on doing so, make sure you use nothing but birdseed, as offering human food is definitely frowned upon as being detrimental to the long-term health of the birds.

Meadows backdropped by Mount Rose and Slide Mountain are close at hand. Upon thoroughly enjoying the beautiful vistas, retrace your steps to the trailhead [1].

MILESTONES

1: Start at trailhead; 2: Chickadee Ridge; 3: Peak 9225; 1: Return to trailhead.

GO GREEN | The Great Basin Institute is involved in outdoor community programs and education. They also provide volunteer opportunities in conjunction with the Galena Creek Visitor Center. Check out their website at www .galenacreekvisitorcenter.org.

OPTIONS | You can vary the return to the car by dropping steeply off the ridge to the lower end of Tahoe Meadows and then proceeding gently uphill back to the highway.

WARM-UPS | The Wildflower Café in Incline Village (869 Tahoe Boulevard) has been feeding locals and tourists fine food for breakfast and lunch for over thirty years. You can see their menus at www.wildflowercafetahoe.com.

22 | Tahoe Viewpoint Loop

This short and easy trip is a fine choice for a morning or afternoon spin around the snow when time is limited or you're searching for a good lake view with minimal effort involved. While hundreds may be cavorting around Tahoe Meadows a short drive away, this route is far less used and offers a chance for solitude, which surely will be lacking in the meadows.

LEVEL	Intermediate
LENGTH	1.8 miles, loop
TIME	Half day
ELEVATION	+275'–275'
DIFFICULTY	Moderate
AVALANCHE RISK	Low
DOGS	OK
FACILITIES	None
MAPS	USGS *Mount Rose*; USFS *Mount Rose Wilderness*
MANAGEMENT	Humboldt-Toiyabe National Forest, Carson Ranger District at 775-882-2766, www.fs.usda.gov/htnf; Lake Tahoe Basin Management Unit at 530-543-2600, www.fs.usda.gov/ltbmu
HIGHLIGHTS	Meadow, scenery, views
LOWLIGHT	Popular

TIP | While the terrain is fairly gentle and the navigation straightforward, the route is almost entirely in the forest, so some route finding is required.

TRAILHEAD | 39°16.968'N, 119°56.058'W Follow the Mount Rose Highway (Nevada State Route 431) to a plowed section of the highway shoulder near a highway gate and electronic sign, 3 miles southwest of Mount Rose Summit.

ROUTE | [1] From the parking area, make a brief ascent of a steep hillside to more level terrain and then traverse through the moderate cover of a

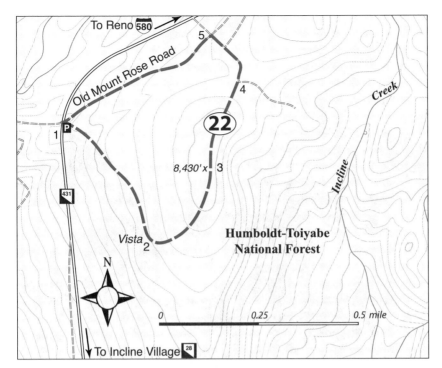

22. Tahoe Viewpoint Loop

lodgepole pine forest to a rock outcropping [2], 0.5 mile from the highway. On top of the outcropping, a beautiful view of Lake Tahoe unfolds.

You could simply retrace your steps to the highway after admiring the view, or follow a loop route instead. Head northeast through the trees to the top of Peak 8430 [3]. From there, proceed north along the ridge to a saddle, where you intersect a snow-covered road [4]. Turn left and follow the road briefly to where it curves to the northeast. Leave the road and follow a northwest course for a short distance to another road [5] paralleling the Mount Rose Highway. Turn left (southwest) and follow this road and an adjacent utility line on a gradually increasing descent. Nearing the highway, the road bends to the right but you proceed ahead, following the route of the utility line back to the parking area [1].

MILESTONES

1: Start at trailhead; 2: Rock outcrop; 3: Top of Peak 8430; 4: Turn left at road; 1: Return to trailhead.

GO GREEN | Snowlands Network is a fine organization dedicated to protecting winter human-powered recreation across public lands. Consult their website at www.snowlands.org.

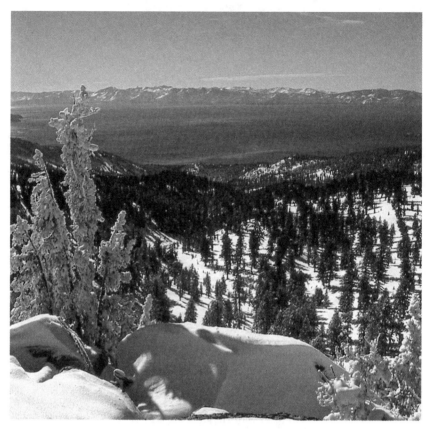

A beautiful view of Lake Tahoe

INCLINE VILLAGE One might rightly wonder about the origin of Incline Village, as the name is anything but common. To fuel the Comstock Lode, almost the entire Lake Tahoe Basin was denuded of timber. But how did all that lumber get to Virginia City? One of the ways involved Incline Village, as a sawmill along nearby Mill Creek was established around 1880. An incline railroad was built to carry lumber from the mill 1,400 vertical feet up the steep hillside above to the banks of Third Creek, where the logs were then sent via a flume for several miles to a tunnel. The tunnel had previously been built beneath the crest of the Carson Range to transport water from Marlette Lake to Virginia City following a devastating fire that destroyed a large portion of the town. A flume was built inside the tunnel above the water level to deliver the lumber to an open flume on the east side of the range to Lakeview, where the Virginia and Truckee Railroad took it the rest of the way to Virginia City.

OPTIONS | There's plenty of snowy terrain nearby for extending your trip if desired.

WARM-UPS | Since its opening in 1981, the Log Cabin Café in Kings Beach (8692 North Lake Boulevard) has been voted more than once as the best place for breakfast in North Tahoe. The small café serves up ample portions of home cooking, with a number of unique dishes (the Cajun Eggs Benedict is a spicy twist on the traditional dish and was featured in *Bon Appétit* magazine). Open seven days a week from 7:00 AM to 2:00 PM, the popular restaurant can be quite busy on weekends. However, the café does allow you to call ahead to be placed on their waiting list (530-546-7109).

PART TWO

EAST TAHOE

The east shore is perhaps the least developed side of Lake Tahoe. Unfortunately, the relative lack of development doesn't necessarily translate into an abundance of routes for snowshoers. The steep topography, composed of the thin spine of the Carson Range rising abruptly from the lakeshore and then plunging just as dramatically toward the valleys of western Nevada, limits the availability of areas suitable for recreational purposes.

Lake Tahoe Nevada State Park administers a fare portion of these limited recreational lands, where volunteers groom cross-country ski tracks and maintain a pair of backcountry cabins. Payment of the park's entrance fee ($7 during winter in 2017, minus $2 discount for Nevada residents), allows snowshoers access to the area, provided they stay out of the cross-country ski tracks.

Some of the land on the east side of Tahoe is unsuitable for backcountry snowshoeing, either due to the presence of snowmobiles or the boundaries of a ski resort. Many human-powered souls may want to avoid these areas. South of Highway 50 near Spooner Summit, a snowmobile concessionaire launches a plethora of motorized vehicles on the slopes toward Daggett Pass, potentially disrupting an otherwise splendid 10-mile tour along the east crest of the Tahoe Basin. Farther south, Heavenly Valley Ski Resort covers the most acreage of any alpine ski area in the Lake Tahoe region.

While the winter terrain on the east side of the lake does have some limiting factors, the few trips included in this guide may provide some of the best snowshoeing in the basin. A spectacular lake view awaits the diligent traveler from the top of Snow Valley Peak on a lightly used route north of Spooner Summit. Inside Lake Tahoe Nevada State Park, the trip to Marlette Lake offers a mildly graded route with pleasant scenery, while the short loop around Spooner Lake is a family favorite.

■ Access

Along with U.S. Highway 50, Nevada State Route 28 provides the principal access to the lands on the east shore of Lake Tahoe. In addition, Kingsbury Grade (State Route 207) is a connector between U.S. 50 at Stateline and the Carson Valley.

■ Communities

While there are no major towns between Incline Village and Stateline, the tiny burgs of Zephyr Cove and Round Hill offer some services to travelers.

**TRIP
23** Lake Tahoe Nevada
State Park

The nearly 2-mile loop around Spooner Lake is a great trip for beginners and families, as the terrain is essentially flat, route finding is straightforward, and the winter scenery is quite pleasant. The minimal distance and gentle terrain combine to make a romp around the lake a good choice for a short morning or afternoon trip.

The journey along the snow-covered North Canyon Road to Marlette Lake offers a fine winter outing for intermediate snowshoers who can handle the nearly 10-mile round-trip distance. Most of the route climbs mildly to moderately on the way to the trip's high point before a half-mile descent leads to the south shore of the very scenic lake.

TRAILHEAD | 39°06.414'N, 119°54.998'W Follow Nevada State Route 28 to the Spooner Lake entrance into Lake Tahoe Nevada State Park, 1 mile northwest of the junction of U.S. 50. Follow the access road past the entrance station (fee) and shortly to the parking area.

A ▪ Spooner Lake	
LEVEL	Novice
LENGTH	2 miles, lollipop loop
TIME	2 hours
ELEVATION	Negligible
DIFFICULTY	Easy
AVALANCHE RISK	Low
DOGS	On leash
FACILITIES	Restrooms
MAP	USGS *Glenbrook*
MANAGEMENT	Lake Tahoe Nevada State Park at 775-831-0494, www.parks.nv.gov/parks/lake-tahoe-nevada-state-park-1
HIGHLIGHT	Lake
LOWLIGHT	Fee

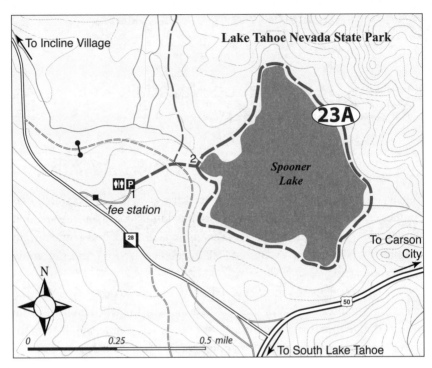

To Incline Village

Lake Tahoe Nevada State Park

23A

Spooner Lake

2

P
1

fee station

28

N

To Carson City

50

To South Lake Tahoe

0   0.25   0.5 mile

23A. Spooner Lake

TIP | Snow conditions can be variable at this elevation. Check with the park about current conditions. Nevada Nordic sets several kilometers of track within the park for cross-country skiers. Snowshoers are welcome to follow these routes but must stay out of the set tracks.

ROUTE | [1] From the parking area, head east toward Spooner Lake. Proceed across the outlet stream and begin a clockwise loop [2] around the lake. If the snowpack is not too deep, you may be able to gain some information about the natural history of the area from several interpretive signs posted around

SPOONER LAKE The lake was created in the 1850s for use as a millpond and the dam was then rebuilt in 1929 for irrigation purposes. Nowadays, recreation has supplanted logging and irrigation as the principal activity within Lake Tahoe Nevada State Park, as people flock to the area in the summer to hike, mountain bike, swim, bird watch, picnic, and fish. A fair number of folks come to the park in winter as well, to cross-country ski or snowshoe.

the lakeshore. A forest of lodgepole pines, white firs, and Jeffrey pines rims the east side of the lake, while a large stand of aspens lines the inlet near the southeast shore. Continue around the lake to complete the loop [2]. From there, retrace your steps to the parking area [1].

MILESTONES

1: Start at trailhead; 2: Start of loop; 2: End of loop; 1: Return to trailhead.

B ▪ Marlette Lake	
LEVEL	Intermediate
LENGTH	9.6 miles, out and back
TIME	Full day
ELEVATION	+1,200'–350'
DIFFICULTY	Moderate to strenuous
AVALANCHE RISK	Low
DOGS	On leash
FACILITIES	Restrooms
MAP	USGS *Glenbrook*
MANAGEMENT	Lake Tahoe Nevada State Park at 775-831-0494, www.parks.nv.gov/parks/lake-tahoe-nevada-state-park-1
HIGHLIGHTS	Forest, lake, scenery
LOWLIGHT	Fee

TIP | The mostly forested route does offer some protection if the day is windy.

ROUTE | [1] From the parking area, follow a wide path for 0.1 mile to access the even broader swath of the North Canyon Road. Head north through open terrain on the way into moderate cover from a mixed forest of Jeffrey and lodgepole pines, and white firs. Stroll past Spencer's Cabin [2] (a good turn-around point for a shorter trip) on your left about a half mile from the parking lot, and then continue uphill along the North Canyon Road for the next 2-plus miles. A short way past the 3-mile mark, a stiffer, three-quarter-mile climb leads to a saddle [3] at the high point of the route.

Head downhill and follow the North Canyon Road to a junction [4] with the Hobart Road above the southeast shore of Marlette Lake. Turn left and follow the road a short distance to the southeast shore [5] where a small peninsula juts into the usually frozen lake. When your time at Marlette Lake comes to an end, retrace your steps to the trailhead [1].

MILESTONES

1: Start at trailhead; 2: Spencer's Cabin; 3: Saddle; 4: Junction of Hobart Road; 5: Marlette Lake; 1: Return to trailhead.

MILESTONES

1: Start at trailhead; 2: Spencer's Cabin; 3: Saddle; 4: Junction of Hobart Road; 5: Marlette Lake; 1: Return to trailhead.

MILESTONES

1: Start at trailhead; 2: Spencer's Cabin; 3: Saddle; 4: Junction of Hobart Road; 5: Marlette Lake; 1: Return to trailhead.

MILESTONES

1: Start at trailhead; 2: Spencer's Cabin; 3: Saddle; 4: Junction of Hobart Road; 5: Marlette Lake; 1: Return to trailhead.

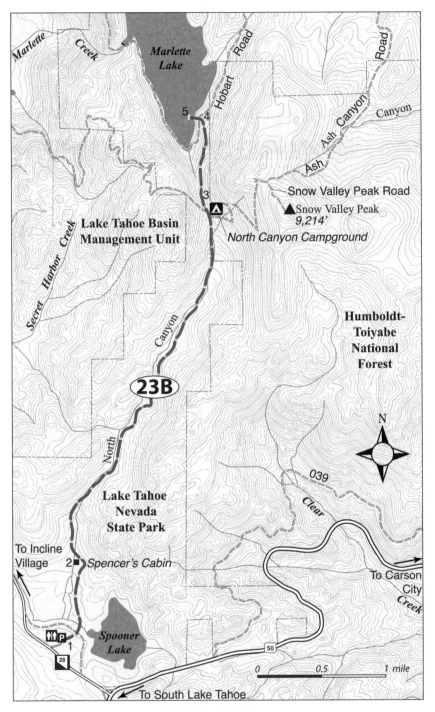

23B. Marlette Lake

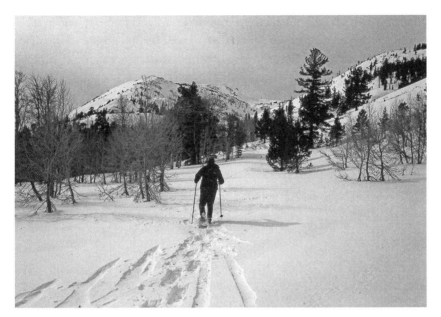

Heading up North Canyon toward Marlette Lake

GO GREEN | Nevada Nordic is a volunteer organization that has adopted the responsibility of setting 10 kilometers of cross-country ski tracks within Lake Tahoe Nevada State Park. Formerly, a concessionaire was responsible for an 80-kilometer trail system within the park, but the multiyear drought seemed to make the enterprise unprofitable. You can assist in this valuable endeavor by donating or offering to volunteer at www.nevadanordic.org.

OPTIONS | Within the park are two Scandinavian-style hand-hewn log cabins for rent, Spooner and Wildcat. The cabins can sleep up to four adults and are equipped with cooking and heating stoves, kitchen supplies, and odor-free composting toilets. Although they were recently only available during the

---

MARLETTE LAKE   The earthen dam that holds back the waters of Marlette Lake was built in 1873 for the purposes of transporting water to Virginia City during the Comstock Lode era. Water from the dam was sent down a flume to Tunnel Creek Station, where the water went through a tunnel beneath the Carson Range and into flumes on the east side of the mountains to Lakeview. From there, an inverted siphon took the water up to Virginia City. Over the years, the dam was raised a number of times until reaching a height of 45 feet in 1959. Marlette Lake and the neighboring land was bought by the State of Nevada in 1963.

summer months, park officials hope the cabins will become open once again during the winter months. Consult the park's website for current information. Formerly, Zephyr Cove Resort was in charge of the rental cabins.

WARM-UPS | Along with winter lodging, Zephyr Cove Resort on the east shore of Lake Tahoe offers dining in the Zephyr Cove Restaurant, complete with lake views and a large stone fireplace to help keep you warm after a spin in the backcountry. Breakfast, lunch, and dinner are served daily. Although the old-fashioned milkshakes here are legendary, a hot beverage from the Zephyr Cove Coffee Bar is certain to take the chill away. Visit their website at www.zephyrcove.com for more information.

TRIP
24 | Snow Valley Peak

Scenic beauty, reasonably dependable weather, and a location close to millions of people combine to make Lake Tahoe a popular winter playground, which makes finding a snowshoe or ski trip offering a fair expectation of solitude oftentimes difficult, especially on a sunny weekend. This route to Snow Valley Peak, loosely following a section of the famed Tahoe Rim Trail, may prove to be just the right ticket for escaping the masses. The price of that ticket, however, is a fairly strenuous trip requiring considerable navigational abilities. Over the first 3 miles, you must negotiate your way through dense forest without the aid of a marked trail or any discernible landmarks. As the trail receives light use, you may not have the benefit of someone else's tracks to follow, either. Therefore, this is a trip for experienced snowshoers only.

Although most of the trip is viewless until near the end, the climax vista from Snow Valley Peak is one of the most spectacular in the Tahoe Basin. From the 9,214-foot summit, the entire lake lies at your feet, and the basin-and-range topography of western Nevada sprawls out to the east.

LEVEL	Advanced
LENGTH	9.6 miles, out and back
TIME	Full day
ELEVATION	+ 2,450'–450'
DIFFICULTY	Strenuous
AVALANCHE RISK	Low to moderate
DOGS	OK
FACILITIES	None
MAPS	USGS *Glenbrook*, *Marlette Lake*
MANAGEMENT	Lake Tahoe Basin Management Unit at 530-543-2600, www.fs.usda.gov/ltbmu
HIGHLIGHTS	Forest, summit, views
LOWLIGHT	Route finding

TIP | A good topographic map, a working compass, a GPS unit with extra batteries, and the skill to use these tools are absolutely essential on this trip.

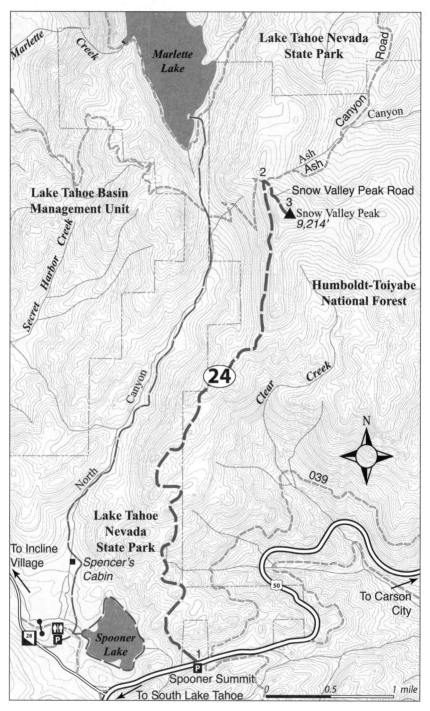

Marlette Creek

Marlette Lake

Lake Tahoe Nevada State Park

Canyon Road

Canyon

Canyon

Ash

Ash

2

Lake Tahoe Basin Management Unit

Snow Valley Peak Road

3 Snow Valley Peak 9,214'

Humboldt-Toiyabe National Forest

Secret Harbor Creek

Canyon

24

Clear Creek

N

North

039

Lake Tahoe Nevada State Park

To Incline Village

Spencer's Cabin

28

P

Spooner Lake

50

To Carson City

1

P

Spooner Summit

To South Lake Tahoe

0   0.5   1 mile

24. Snow Valley Peak

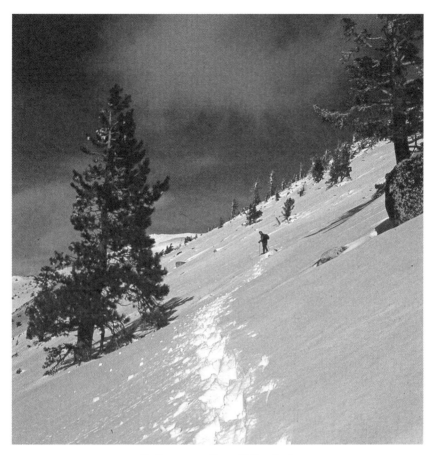

On the way to Snow Valley Peak

TRAILHEAD | 39°06.260'N, 119°53.830'W Follow U.S. Highway 50 to the Tahoe Rim Trail parking area, 0.75 mile east of the junction of Nevada State Route 28 and 9 miles west of the junction of U.S. Highway 395 in Carson City. Park your vehicle in the plowed area on the north shoulder of the highway.

ROUTE | [1] The best path would be to follow the Tahoe Rim Trail all the way to Snow Valley Peak, but doing so without the aid of a marked trail would be difficult unless you're very familiar with the route. After a short climb away from the highway, you follow a slightly ascending traverse across the hillsides above Spooner Lake far below. Once beyond the vicinity of the lake, climb more moderately along a northerly compass bearing through dense forest, as you work your way toward the ridge crest above North Canyon immediately to the west.

While not impossible, finding the most efficient way over and around the various buttes and high points along the ridge is made difficult by the thick woodland. Due to the infrequent use of this route, chances are you won't have much assistance from the tracks of previous visitors. Although some elevation loss is inevitable en route, minimize the amount while maintaining a general ascent in a northeasterly direction. Rarely, the trees may thin just enough to allow fleeting glimpses of Lake Tahoe to the west, or Eagle Valley to the east, which may allow you to momentarily gain your bearings.

After 3 miles through a mixed forest of pines and firs, you arrive at the base of the long ridge leading to the top of Snow Valley Peak. Turning north, you make an angling upward ascent of the west slope of this ridge, as the trees finally begin to thin. The miles of viewless slog are soon forgotten, as a panoramic view of Lake Tahoe unfolds. Above the far shore, the waters of Emerald Bay and Fallen Leaf Lake sparkle below the snow-covered peaks of Desolation Wilderness. Continue the long upward trek across moderately steep slopes on the way to a saddle [2] between Snow Valley Peak and an unnamed peak to the north.

From the saddle, turn southeast and ascend the final slope to the summit [3], where a truly awe-inspiring view awaits. Arriving in pleasant weather should allow you to spy cross-country skiers in the canyon below on their way to and from Marlette Lake. Packing along a small-scale map will help you identify the numerous Tahoe landmarks visible from this stunning aerie. After thoroughly enjoying the view, retrace your steps to the trailhead [1].

MILESTONES
1: Start at TRT trailhead; 2: Saddle; 3: Summit of Snow Valley Peak; 1: Return to trailhead.

> QUAKING ASPEN (*Populus tremuloides*) Once the trees part enough to allow views down into North Canyon and Marlette Lake, you may notice a preponderance of quaking aspens lining the stream and lake. Brilliant gold in autumn and yellow-green in summer, even in winter the bare limbs of these trees are distinctive. Although growing from seeds is possible, most aspens sprout from the spreading roots of a single parent, amazingly resulting in stands of genetically identical individuals.

GO GREEN | You can support conservation of the north Tahoe region by joining the Sierra Club, either through the Toiyabe (sierraclub.org/toiyabe) or Mother Lode (sierraclub.org/mother-lode) Chapters.

OPTIONS | Those possessed with plenty of extra energy could vary their return to the trailhead on a loop route that descends from the saddle [2] on the zigzagging course of the Snow Valley Road down to North Canyon Road. From there, head south and then southwest down the canyon to Spooner Lake. Climb the slope above the southeast shore back to the parking area [1].

WARM-UPS | Along with winter lodging, Zephyr Cove Resort on the east shore of Lake Tahoe offers dining in the Zephyr Cove Restaurant, complete with lake views and a large stone fireplace to help warm you up after a spin in the backcountry. Breakfast, lunch, and dinner are served daily. Although the old-fashioned milkshakes here are legendary, a hot beverage from the Zephyr Cove Coffee Bar is certain to take the chill away. Visit their website at www.zephyrcove.com for more information.

TRIP
25 Castle Rock

This short trip would garner an easy rating if not for the final scramble necessary to reach the top of Castle Rock for the inspiring Lake Tahoe vista. Requiring only a slight bit of navigation, the mostly forested route briefly follows the course of a snow-covered jeep road down the drainage of Burke Creek to a rising traverse up to a minor saddle, followed by a short, moderate climb to the base of Castle Rock. Even in summer getting to the top demands technical climbing skills. However, a less ambitious scramble of the slightly lower pinnacle to the south will reward you with an equally impressive view of Lake Tahoe. Although the distance is short and the navigation fairly straightforward to the base of Castle Rock, the scramble is over steep snow ramps and moderate-angle rock slabs, which makes the finale for the experienced only. Less brave souls can still revel in a fine view of the lake and Carson Valley to the east from the base of Castle Rock.

LEVEL	Intermediate
LENGTH	2.5 miles, out and back
TIME	Half day
ELEVATION	+275'–250'
DIFFICULTY	Moderate
DOGS	OK
FACILITIES	None
MAP	USGS *South Lake Tahoe*
MANAGEMENT	Lake Tahoe Basin Management Unit at 530-543-2600, www.fs.usda.gov/ltbmu
HIGHLIGHT	Views
LOWLIGHTS	Limited parking, snowmobiles

TIP | The Genoa Peak Road is a favorite haunt of snowmobilers. You can minimize the exposure to the noise and exhaust from these machines by taking this trip on a weekday, when the traffic may be considerably less.

TRAILHEAD | 38°59.691'N, 119°53.794'W Follow Highway 207 (Kingsbury Grade) to North Benjamin Drive (2.9 miles eastbound from Highway 50 and 0.3 mile westbound of Daggett Pass). Turn north and follow North Benjamin

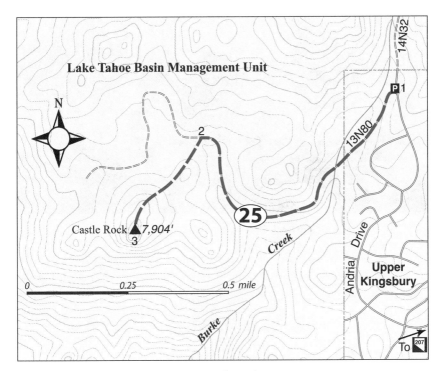

25. Castle Rock

Drive, which soon becomes Andria Road, to the end of plowed road, 1.75 miles from the highway. Park on the shoulder as space allows, obeying the sign to stay out of the snowplow turnaround.

ROUTE | [1] From the parking area, parallel the road for a short distance to where Forest Service Road 13N80 heads downhill through the drainage of Burke Creek on a moderate descent through a mixed forest of Jeffrey pines, lodgepole pines, and white firs. After a half mile, make a slightly rising traverse around the base of a hill on your right to a broad, forested saddle [2] northeast of Castle Rock.

A mile from the trailhead, you head away from the saddle on a southwest course, climbing moderately toward Castle Rock past a subsidiary knob to your left along the way. The grade increases even more on the approach to the base of the rock, where the forest cover blocks any possible views of the lake.

Reaching the true summit of Castle Rock requires technical climbing skills. However, unobstructed views of Lake Tahoe are available from the slightly lower pinnacle [3] to the south via a slightly less daunting scramble up snow ramps and slabs. Successful summiteers will revel in a spectacular Tahoe view, including Marla Bay just to the right of Round Hill and the Crystal Range peaks glistening in the sun above the far shore. For those intimidated

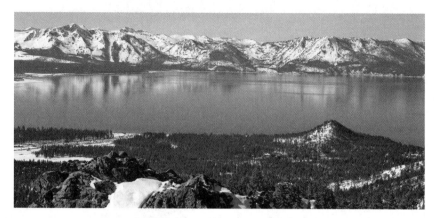

Castle Rock offers grand Lake Tahoe views.

by the scramble, views of the lake may be attainable from the west base of the rock, as well as views of Carson Valley from the east side. After admiring the view, retrace your steps to the trailhead [1].

DAGGETT PASS The pass was named for Charles D. Daggett, who settled on a ranch in western Carson Valley in 1854 and was one of the few doctors in the area. The Daggett Trail was a foot and horse route that connected the valley to the southeast shore of Lake Bigler (Tahoe). In the mid-1800s, David D. Kingsbury and John McDonald advanced the route and opened a toll road ultimately used by the Pony Express and then the Overland Stage Line. The modern highway follows an improved alignment of the route but crosses the old road at several locations.

MILESTONES

1: Start at parking area; 2: Forested saddle; 3: Castle Rock; 1: Return to parking area.

GO GREEN | Snowlands Network is a fine organization dedicated to protecting winter human-powered recreation across public lands. Consult their website at www.snowlands.org.

OPTIONS | Plenty of backcountry lies to the north of Castle Rock, but be prepared for some navigation if you choose to head in that direction.

WARM-UPS | The Red Hut Café at 229 Kingsbury Grade is a fine place to dine before or after a jaunt to Castle Rock. The restaurant is open seven days a week from 6:00 AM to 2:00 PM, serving ample portions of inexpensive diner fare. Visit their website at www.redhutcafe.com for more information.

PART THREE

SOUTH TAHOE

To some, mention of the south shore of Lake Tahoe conjures up visions of opulent hotel-casinos, excessive commercialism, and traffic jams, which is perhaps an accurate portrayal of some of the area. However, beyond the excessive visual stimulation, crush of tourists, and the accompanying din, the backcountry beyond this end of the lake is possibly the most dramatic and inspiring section of topography in Northern California. Certainly, had history unfolded differently and there had been no Comstock Lode, a Lake Tahoe National Park would seem to be a reasonable possibility. The spectacular mountain scenery around the southern reaches of the lake would have provided a profound punctuation point for just such a preserve. Whether you're searching for rugged peaks, incomparable vistas, serene meadows, or challenging ascents, the south Tahoe region won't disappoint any lover of mountains.

South Tahoe as described in the guide encompasses the landscape around some of the highest mountain passes in the area—Carson Pass, Luther Pass, and Echo Summit. The relatively high elevations near these passes provide access to some of the best snow conditions in the greater Lake Tahoe region. This arbitrary delineation also includes the topography around Fallen Leaf Lake, with access primarily from the south due to periodic closures of State Route 89 around Emerald Bay for avalanche control. Some of Tahoe's highest peaks and most mountainous topography are here as well, found within two federally designated wilderness areas, Desolation and Mokelumne.

Due to the rugged terrain, many of the trips in this chapter are rated as moderate or difficult. However, a few trips (Scotts Lake, Big Meadow, Angora Lookout, and Fallen Leaf Lake) do have an easy rating or have easy sections suitable for beginning snowshoers. At the other end of the spectrum, some of the summits mentioned (Mount Tallac, Waterhouse Peak, and Thompson Peak) should provide significant challenges for even the most experienced and fit snowshoers. Several additional trips fill in the middle ground.

Carson Pass, Meiss Meadows, Echo Lakes, and Taylor Creek SNO-PARKS provide developed access and parking for a number of trips described in this chapter. Other trailheads may have extremely limited parking opportunities, some of which may necessitate creative solutions. Planning trips for the middle of the week may limit some of the parking difficulties.

■ Access

U.S. 50 is the major arterial along the south shore of Lake Tahoe. California State Route 89 meets U.S. 50 at the Y in South Lake Tahoe and then continues southbound through Meyers, over Luther Pass, and down to State Route 88 at Picketts Junction. State Route 88 connects the Nevada communities of Minden and Gardnerville to California's Gold Country.

■ Communities

The south end of Lake Tahoe harbors the area's largest population at South Lake Tahoe. Spanning the gamut from high-end casinos to greasy spoons, this side of Tahoe offers plenty of services to the traveler.

TRIP 26
High Meadows and Star Lake

High Meadows is a picturesque clearing beyond the southeast shore of Lake Tahoe in the shadow of 10,881-foot Freel Peak (the Tahoe Basin's highest mountain) and 10,823-foot Jobs Sister. Before the relatively recent construction of the Tahoe Rim Trail, the dirt road to High Meadows provided the sole access to isolated and lovely Star Lake. Unfortunately, that road was on private land and off-limits to the public until 2003.

The road to High Meadows is moderately graded and easy to follow, providing snowshoers and skiers a straightforward route through dense forest to a series of clearings along Cold Creek. The meadows provide an excellent destination for parties seeking a relatively short (three and one-quarter miles) trip with minimal elevation gain (1,250 feet), requiring only basic route-finding skills.

The longer route to Star Lake is a more difficult and strenuous proposition. Along with the greater distance and elevation gain, advanced route-finding skills will be necessary beyond High Meadows in order to successfully reach the lake. The fantastic scenery will reward those who do, with a frozen lake cradled into an impressive cirque and backdropped by the imposing north face of Jobs Sister.

LEVEL	Intermediate (High Meadows); advanced (Star Lake)
LENGTH	6.5 miles, out and back (High Meadows); 11 miles, out and back (Star Lake)
TIME	Three-quarter day (High Meadows); full day (Star Lake)
ELEVATION	+1,400'–200' (High Meadows); +2,650'–200' (Star Lake)
DIFFICULTY	Moderate (High Meadows); strenuous (Star Lake)
AVALANCHE RISK	Low to moderate
DOGS	OK
FACILITIES	None
MAP	USGS *South Lake Tahoe*
MANAGEMENT	Lake Tahoe Basin Management Unit at 530-543-2600, www.fs.usda.gov/ltbmu
HIGHLIGHTS	Forest, lake, meadows, scenery
LOWLIGHT	Route finding

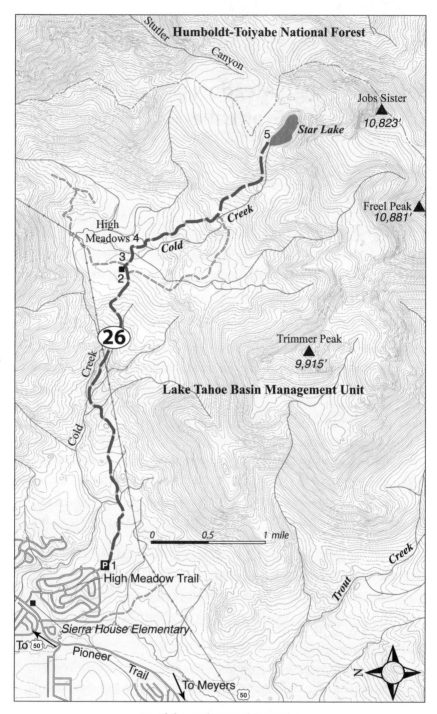

26. High Meadows and Star Lake

THE GIOVACCHINI FAMILY Permanent residents of Carson Valley, the Giovacchinis sold a 1,790-acre parcel of their south Tahoe holdings to the Forest Service via the American Land Conservancy in 2003. Nowadays, visitors in any season can legally travel their old road to High Meadows and continue to Star Lake beyond. They retained 490 acres near the meadows, but an easement allows the public to cross their property via the road. Therefore, stay on the route of the road as best you can while traveling in winter.

TIP | Snow conditions may be variable at the beginning of this trip. Walking along the road for a stretch may be necessary to reach sufficient snow depth for snowshoes, particularly as spring approaches.

TRAILHEAD | 38°53.876'N, 119°57.455'W From U.S. 50 in South Lake Tahoe, follow Pioneer Trail for 3.3 miles (or 4.5 miles from 50/89 in Meyers) to the vicinity of Sierra House Elementary School and turn southeast onto High Meadows Trail. Drive 0.7 mile to the end of the plowed section of road and park your vehicle as space allows.

ROUTE | [1] Follow the continuation of the road on a very mild climb through mixed forest. Cross a wooden bridge spanning a tributary of Cold Creek at three-quarters of a mile, pass by a ramshackle cabin, and then start climbing a little more steeply beyond a small meadow. The road follows the course of a utility line for a while before ascending to the top of a forested flat. From there, make a short drop to a pair of crossings of Cold Creek at 1.6 and 1.7 miles. Beyond the creek crossings, make a steady climb up the nose of a forested ridge between twin channels of the creek. As you progress up the hillside, the forest parts just enough to allow a momentary view of the south end of Lake Tahoe and some of the peaks in Desolation Wilderness. Veer to the right where a secondary road travels along a power line cut and proceed to a Y-junction [2] at 3 miles from the trailhead.

Bear left at the junction and continue along the road past an old cabin. About 25 yards farther is a T-junction [3] where you turn right, soon coming to the west edge of High Meadows [4]. If you are not going any farther, after exploring the meadows retrace your steps to the trailhead [1].

Continuing to Star Lake, the exact course of the road is hard to determine in the open meadows, although, technically, it does proceed to a crossing of the aspen-lined creek near the south end. As both the course of the road and the route of the summer hiking trail farther on tend to become very difficult to discern, simply head east briefly and then turn upstream to follow the course of Cold Creek. Head up the left-hand side of the canyon through mixed forest with occasional Tahoe views behind. Continue steadily ascending up the canyon until reaching the west shore of beautiful Star Lake [5], nestled into a picturesque cirque below the towering north face of Jobs Sister. When the time comes, retrace your steps to the trailhead [1].

MILESTONES

1: Start at trailhead; 2: Left at Y-junction; 3: Right at T-junction; 4: High Meadows; 5: Star Lake; 1: Return to trailhead.

GO GREEN | The American Land Conservancy, which helped broker the deal to open this area to the public, is now defunct. However, you can support similar efforts in the Lake Tahoe area through the Tahoe Fund. Visit their website at www.tahoefund.org.

OPTIONS | The full-day trip to Star Lake should be enough of an effort for the most hardy of snowshoers.

WARM-UPS | The Red Hut Café has three locations in South Tahoe, a new version at 3660 Lake Tahoe Boulevard (corner of U.S. 50 and Ski Run Boulevard), the original restaurant that opened in 1959 at 2723 Lake Tahoe Boulevard, and one at 229 Kingsbury Grade. The two older restaurants are open seven days a week from 6 AM to 2:00 PM, but the newer one stays open for dinner as well. Any of the three would be a solid place to stop for breakfast on your way to the trailhead for ample portions of inexpensive diner fare. Visit their website at www.redhutcafe.com for more information.

TRIP

27 | Big Meadow

Striding across the smooth surface of the snow carpeting Big Meadow while enjoying the delightful scenery is a grand way to spend part of a morning or afternoon, particularly for beginning snowshoers. The area is also a fine spot for more experienced users searching for a mellow way to ease into the winter season, or for those who only have a couple of hours to spare. The initial ascent up to the meadow is quickly forgotten where the grade eases and the open terrain reveals the splendid setting of the clearing rimmed by evergreen forest.

LEVEL	Novice
LENGTH	1.8 miles, lollipop loop
TIME	2 hours
ELEVATION	+350'–0'
DIFFICULTY	Easy
AVALANCHE RISK	Low
DOGS	OK
FACILITIES	None
MAPS	USGS *Echo Lake, Freel Peak*
MANAGEMENT	Lake Tahoe Basin Management Unit at 530-543-2600, www.fs.usda.gov/ltbmu
HIGHLIGHTS	Forest, meadow
LOWLIGHT	Parking

TIP | As parking is very limited, try to arrive early on weekends to secure a spot.

TRAILHEAD | 38°47.216'N, 120°00.110'W Drive on California State Route 89 to the vicinity of the Tahoe Rim Trail summer trailhead, 3.3 miles west of Luther Pass and 5 miles from the junction of U.S. 50 near Meyers. A small plowed parking area on the north shoulder of the highway is across from the trailhead.

ROUTE | [1] From State Route 89, climb moderately through a forest of pines and firs up the drainage of Big Meadow Creek, staying well above the

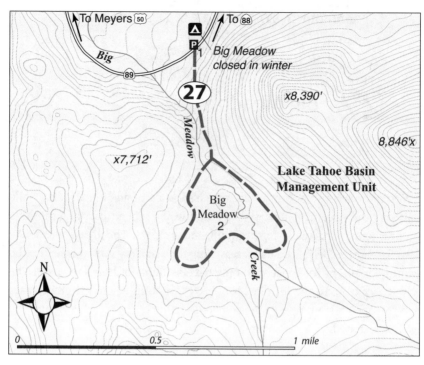

27. Big Meadow

aspen-lined stream to your right. Weave around through the trees in the drainage, heading for the broad expanse of Big Meadow above. After about a half mile, the grade gradually eases just before you reach the meadow. Aptly named Big Meadow [2] is a beautiful setting, surrounded by dense forest and bisected by the creek. Beyond the far edge of the clearing, rugged-looking Waterhouse Peak rises above the surrounding topography (see Map 28). Looping around the large meadow may require negotiating a route across Big Meadow Creek. When your time is up, retrace your steps to the trailhead [1].

WATERMELON SNOW (*Chlamydomonas nivalis*) After mid-March, temperatures usually begin to rise as winter gives way to spring in the Sierra and the accumulated snowfall begins the long melting process. In sunny areas you may notice a pink stain on snowbanks, which is created by the presence of algae. These tiny organisms are actually green in color but secrete carotenoid pigment as a covering for protection from the intense solar radiation. Don't eat any of this discolored snow, as it may act as a strong laxative in some humans.

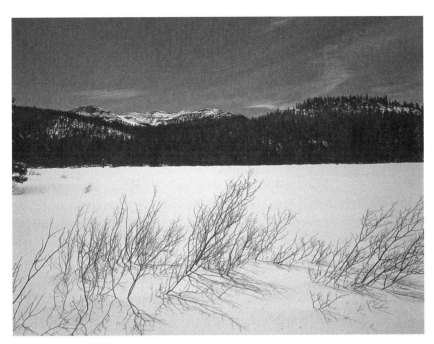

Winter serenity at Big Meadow

MILESTONES
1: Start at trailhead; 2: Big Meadow; 1: Return to trailhead.

GO GREEN | Snowlands Network is a fine organization dedicated to protecting winter human-powered recreation across public lands. Consult their website at www.snowlands.org.

OPTIONS | For a greater challenge on a longer excursion, check out the following trips beyond Big Meadow to Scotts Lake (Trip 28) or Round Lake (Trip 29).

WARM-UPS | Located at 2279 Lake Tahoe Boulevard #2 in South Lake Tahoe, Keys Café is an independent coffeehouse, restaurant, wine and dessert bar, and Internet café open every day from 7:00 AM to 4:00 PM. The establishment occupies a cozy cabin and serves specialty breakfast items, as well as salads, soups, wraps, and sandwiches for lunch. For more information, visit their website at www.tahoekeyscafe.com.

28 Big Meadow to Scotts Lake

Enjoy a large meadow, a good-size lake, and some excellent views of the Hope Valley and Carson Pass areas. The route follows Big Meadow Creek to Big Meadow and then climbs to an 8,000-foot pass before shortly dropping to Scotts Lake. Basic route-finding skills are required to navigate through the forested terrain, but for those desiring to expand such skills, the straightforward nature of the topography on this trip provides a reasonably direct way to transition from marked trails to cross-country travel.

LEVEL	Intermediate
LENGTH	6 miles, out and back
TIME	Three-quarter day
ELEVATION	+900'–175'
DIFFICULTY	Moderate
AVALANCHE RISK	Low
DOGS	OK
FACILITIES	None
MAPS	USGS *Echo Lake*, *Freel Peak*
MANAGEMENT	Lake Tahoe Basin Management Unit at 530-543-2600, www.fs.usda.gov/ltbmu; Humboldt-Toiyabe National Forest at 775-882-2766, www.fs.usda.gov/htnf
HIGHLIGHTS	Forest, lake, meadow, views
LOWLIGHT	Parking

TIP | As parking is very limited, try to arrive early on weekends to secure a spot.

TRAILHEAD | 38°47.216'N, 120°00.110'W Drive on California State Route 89 to the vicinity of the Tahoe Rim Trail summer trailhead, 3.3 miles west of Luther Pass and 5 miles from the junction of U.S. 50 near Meyers. A small plowed parking area on the north shoulder of the highway is across from the trailhead.

ROUTE | [1] The initial part of the route is the same as in Trip 27 toward Big Meadow. From State Route 89, climb moderately through a forest of pines and

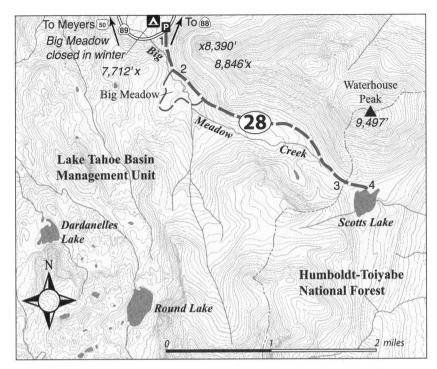

28. Big Meadow to Scotts Lake

firs up the drainage of Big Meadow Creek, staying well above the aspen-lined stream to your right. Weave around through the trees in the drainage, heading for the broad expanse of Big Meadow above. After about half a mile, the grade gradually eases just before you reach the meadow. Aptly named Big Meadow [2] is a beautiful setting, surrounded by dense forest and bisected by the creek. Beyond the far edge of the clearing, rugged-looking Waterhouse Peak rises above the surrounding topography.

Head southeast through Big Meadow and then follow above the left-hand bank of Big Meadow Creek up the heavily forested upper canyon. Stay a good distance up the side of the canyon, as the creek bottom is full of timber, deadfalls, and brush. Continue the ascent through the trees toward the head of the canyon. Approaching a saddle, the grade eases and the trees start to thin enough to allow momentary views of Waterhouse Peak and the ridge on the opposite side of the canyon. Reach the 8,080-foot pass [3] at 2.7 miles from the highway, which sits on a ridge dividing the drainages of the Upper Truckee River behind you and the West Fork Carson River ahead. Beautiful views from the pass include the northeast face of Stevens Peak to the west.

Just below the saddle lie the frozen waters of Scotts Lake [4], picturesquely located below the steep flank of Stevens Peak. The enjoyable setting

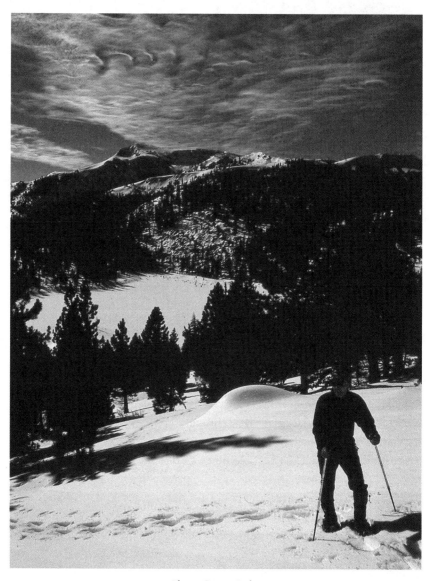

Above Scotts Lake

is a fine location for an extended break or lunch spot. After soaking in the beautiful surroundings, retrace your steps to the trailhead [1].

MILESTONES

1: Start at trailhead; 2: Big Meadow; 3: Saddle; 4: Scotts Lake; 1: Return to trailhead.

GO GREEN | The Tahoe Fund advocates for conservation of the Lake Tahoe Basin. You can visit their website at www.tahoefund.org to learn about their mission and projects.

> **WATERHOUSE PEAK** The 9,497-foot peak directly north of Scotts Lake was named in memory of Clark Waterhouse. After being in charge of the Angora Lookout, he died in World War I. The mountain is a favorite among the backcountry ski and board crowd.

OPTIONS | Ambitious snowshoers with extra energy could elect to scale Waterhouse Peak from the saddle for a fantastic view of the surrounding terrain.

WARM-UPS | Now housed in the renovated shopping center near the base of Heavenly Valley's tram in South Lake (1001 Heavenly Village Way), Bud and Michelle Hillman's family-friendly Driftwood Café has been serving interesting, atypical breakfast and lunch cuisine from 7:00 AM to 3:00 PM daily since 1999. Visit their website at www.driftwoodtahoe.com.

29 | Round Lake

When a fresh blanket of snow carpets the environs around Round Lake, a setting more picturesque is hard to imagine. The circular lake is cradled beneath the striking cliffs of the Dardanelles, a volcanic formation that glistens in the winter sunlight after a dusting of light snow. Add in the trip through Big Meadow and a fine view of the Upper Truckee River drainage from the trip's high point and you have an unbeatable choice for a winter outing.

LEVEL	Intermediate
LENGTH	5.6 miles, out and back
TIME	Three-quarter day
ELEVATION	+700'–675'
DIFFICULTY	Moderate
AVALANCHE RISK	Low to moderate
DOGS	OK
FACILITIES	None
MAPS	USGS *Echo Lake*, *Freel Peak*
MANAGEMENT	Lake Tahoe Basin Management Unit at 530-543-2600, www.fs.usda.gov/ltbmu; Humboldt-Toiyabe National Forest at 775-882-2766, www.fs.usda.gov/htnf
HIGHLIGHTS	Forest, lake, meadow, views
LOWLIGHT	Parking

TIP | As parking is very limited, try to arrive early on weekends to secure a spot.

TRAILHEAD | 38°47.216'N, 120°00.110'W Drive on California State Route 89 to the vicinity of the Tahoe Rim Trail summer trailhead, 3.3 miles west of Luther Pass and 5 miles from the junction of U.S. 50 near Meyers. A small plowed parking area on the north shoulder of the highway is across from the trailhead.

ROUTE | [1] The initial part of the route is the same as in Trip 27 toward Big Meadow and Trip 28 to Scotts Lake. From State Route 89, climb moderately through a forest of pines and firs up the drainage of Big Meadow Creek, staying

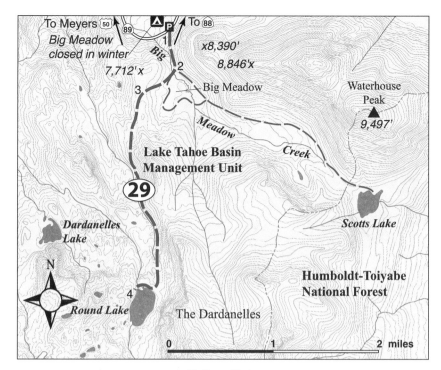

29. Round Lake

well above the aspen-lined stream to your right. Weave around through the trees in the drainage, heading for the broad expanse of Big Meadow above. After about a half mile, the grade gradually eases just before you reach the meadow. Aptly named Big Meadow [2] is a beautiful setting, surrounded by dense forest and bisected by the creek. Beyond the far edge of the clearing, rugged-looking Waterhouse Peak rises above the surrounding topography.

From the near edge of Big Meadow, travel south across the meadow. After entering a covering of moderate forest, continue to bear south on a gradual ascent of the ridge west of the west branch of Big Meadow Creek. The grade increases as you draw near a forested pinnacle, a half mile from Big Meadow. Pass below the pinnacle across the forested slopes on the east flank of the ridge and continue the ascent through lighter forest cover up to a pass [3] on a ridge dividing the tributaries of Big Meadow Creek and the Upper Truckee River, 1.7 miles from the trailhead. At the pass are good views of Waterhouse Peak and the surrounding terrain. The view of the Upper Truckee River country is quite impressive as well.

From the pass, make an angling descent across the steep hillside down to the bottom of the forested drainage. Then proceed up the canyon, working your way over to the main channel of the creek draining Round Lake. Following the creek, you eventually reach a steep slope just before the lake. Once

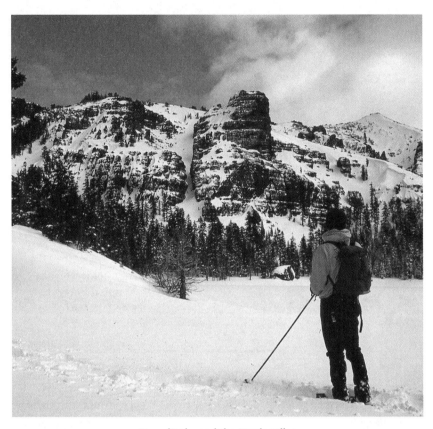

Round Lake and the Dardanelles

you've surmounted this final incline, descend shortly to the north shore of lovely Round Lake [4].

Round Lake is located in an extraordinarily beautiful setting, under the sheer volcanic cliffs above the east shore known as the Dardanelles. After enjoying the lovely surroundings, retrace your steps to the trailhead [1].

MILESTONES

1: Start at trailhead; 2: Big Meadow; 3: Pass; 4: Round Lake; 1: Return to trailhead.

GO GREEN | You can support conservation of the greater Tahoe region by joining the Sierra Club, either through the Toiyabe (sierraclub.org/toiyabe) or Mother Lode (sierraclub.org/mother-lode) Chapters.

OPTIONS | For a straightforward trip extension, you could climb an additional 300 vertical feet in one and one-quarter miles to visit Meiss Lake (*Caples Lake* map would be necessary). A car shuttle would avoid backtracking and allow for an 8-plus-mile trip between Big Meadow and the Meiss Meadow SNO-PARK on State Route 88 (see Trip 37).

> **THE DARDANELLES** Although the origin is unconfirmed, speculation indicates that these volcanic cliffs above the east shore of Round Lake were possibly named by the Whitney Survey for their resemblance to the mountain castles standing guard over a narrow strait connecting the Sea of Marmara in northwestern Turkey and southeastern Greece to the Aegean Sea at the boundary between Europe and Asia.

WARM-UPS | The Red Hut Café has three locations in South Tahoe, a new version at 3660 Lake Tahoe Boulevard (corner of U.S. 50 and Ski Run Boulevard), the original restaurant that opened in 1959 at 2723 Lake Tahoe Boulevard, and one at 229 Kingsbury Grade. The two older restaurants are open seven days a week from 6:00 AM to 2:00 PM, but the newer one stays open for dinner as well. Any of the three would be a solid place to stop for breakfast on your way to the trailhead for ample portions of inexpensive diner fare. Visit their website at www.redhutcafe.com for more information.

30 | Grass Lake Meadow

The Grass Lake area is a fine place for beginners to acquire a feel for the sport of snowshoeing. The flat terrain is easily negotiated and the openness of the meadow does not demand hardly any navigational skills. Situated below the northeast slope of Waterhouse Peak, the meadow is an attractive winter locale and would be an equally fine destination for more experienced snowshoers in search of a short and easy spin around the snow.

LEVEL Novice

LENGTH Varies, .5 mile to 3.8 miles

TIME 1 hour to half day

ELEVATION Negligible

DIFFICULTY Easy

AVALANCHE RISK Low

DOGS OK

FACILITIES None

MAP USGS *Freel Peak*

MANAGEMENT Lake Tahoe Basin Management Unit at 530-543-2600, www.fs.usda.gov/ltbmu; Humboldt-Toiyabe National Forest at 775-882-2766, www.fs.usda.gov/htnf

HIGHLIGHTS Meadow, scenery

LOWLIGHT None

TIP | Parking may be limited on sunny weekends, so arrive early to secure a space.

TRAILHEAD | 38°47.346'N, 119°56.879'W Drive on California State Route 89 south from South Lake Tahoe, or north from the junction of State Route 88 to Luther Pass. Park your vehicle in the plowed area near the pass along the highway shoulder.

ROUTE | Ascend the snowbank at the edge of the parking area and stroll about the meadow in whatever direction you feel led. A small lobe of the meadow

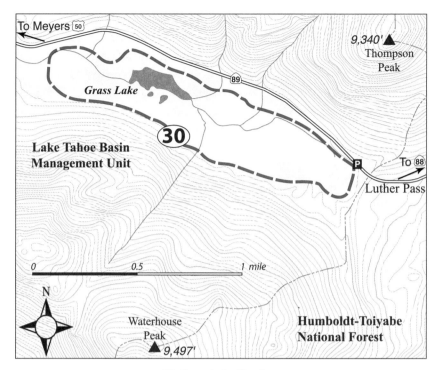

30. Grass Lake Meadow

at the east end near Luther Pass is separated by a grove of trees from the much larger main section. A complete loop around the entire perimeter of the meadow is not quite 4 miles long.

GO GREEN | Snowlands Network is a fine organization dedicated to protecting winter human-powered recreation across public lands. Consult their website at www.snowlands.org.

OPTIONS | An extra challenge for those with extra time and energy would be to scale Waterhouse Peak from the meadow.

IRA MANLEY LUTHER Raised in New York State, Ira Manley Luther (1821–1890), traveled to the west in the 1850s, settling in Sacramento. He crossed his namesake pass sometime later, traveling between Lake and Hope Valleys and painting his name on a rock. He also lived in Nevada for a time on a ranch near Genoa, served in the state legislature for a couple of years, and operated a sawmill near the mouth of Fay Canyon in the 1860s.

Travelers on State Route 88 can dine on fresh-made cuisine at Sorensen's Resort, 0.9 mile east of the 88/89 junction. The charming café with a quaint mountain setting is open each day, serving breakfast from 7:30 AM to 11:00 AM, lunch from 11:00 AM to 4:00 PM, and dinner (reservations advised) from 5:00 PM to 8:30 PM. A variety of lodging is also available, from cozy bed-and-breakfast cottages to log cabins and rental homes. Visit their website at www.sorensensresort.com.

TRIP

31 Thompson Peak

Although the distance from the highway to the summit of Thompson Peak is less than a mile, the terrain is exceedingly steep, gaining 1,600 vertical feet in about three-quarters of a mile. If the snow conditions near the summit are less than ideal, the ascent can be extremely difficult as well. Therefore, the short, steep climb to the summit is recommended for very experienced parties only.

LEVEL	Extreme
LENGTH	1.6 miles, out and back
TIME	Half day
ELEVATION	+1,600'−0'
DIFFICULTY	Very strenuous
AVALANCHE RISK	Moderate to high
DOGS	Not recommended
FACILITIES	None
MAP	USGS *Freel Peak*
MANAGEMENT	Lake Tahoe Basin Management Unit at 530-543-2600, www.fs.usda.gov/ltbmu
HIGHLIGHTS	Summit, views
LOWLIGHT	Very steep

TIP | Due to the steep topography, use only mountaineering-style snowshoes. If the snow is wind packed or hard, an ice axe and crampons might be needed.

TRAILHEAD | 38°47.346'N, 119°56.879'W Drive on California State Route 89 south from South Lake Tahoe, or north from the junction of State Route 88 to Luther Pass. Park your vehicle in the plowed area near the pass along the highway shoulder.

ROUTE | [1] From Luther Pass, begin climbing northeast directly up the steep slope above through a smattering of pines, firs, and quaking aspens. The best line of ascent seems to be to follow just below the ridge crest. Continue to climb as the grade increases and the trees thin on the way to the top. The snow conditions on the upper part of the mountain may affect your mode of

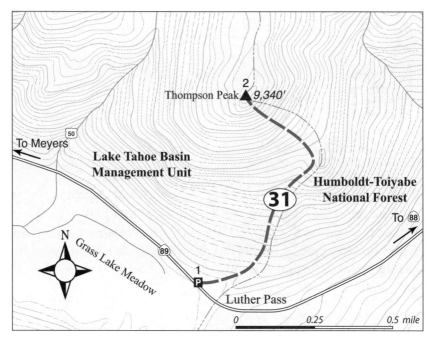

31. Thompson Peak

ascent: if you encounter hardpack snow, removing your snowshoes may make the climb easier to negotiate.

The view from the summit of Thompson Peak is spectacular in all directions. Although Lake Tahoe is out of sight, the vista certainly doesn't lack for inspiring scenery. The peaks around Carson Pass and south Tahoe are almost too numerous to count.

SNOWSHOE THOMPSON, THE FATHER OF CALIFORNIA SKIING Born Jon Torsteinson Rue (1827–1876) in Norway, Thompson came to the United States as a ten-year-old and settled with his family in the Midwest. In 1851, he and his brother drove a herd of milk cows to California, where he lived for nine years before homesteading a ranch south of Genoa in Diamond Valley. From 1856 to 1876, Thompson delivered mail between Placerville and Genoa and later to Virginia City. Despite his nickname, during his winter deliveries he never used snowshoes but instead used 10-foot-long oak skis and a single pole to traverse the Sierra Nevada. His initial trip was done in a mere three days. He preferred to travel mostly at night when the snow was firm and fast. Despite his Herculean feats, he was never paid for his service. His grave resides in the Genoa cemetery.

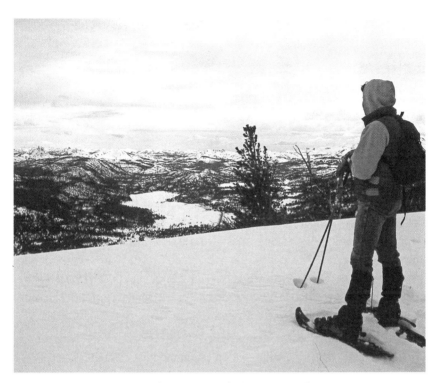

Vista from the top of Thompson Peak

MILESTONES

1: Start at trailhead; 2: Summit of Thompson Peak; 1: Return to trailhead.

GO GREEN | You can help the League to Save Lake Tahoe "Keep Tahoe Blue" by donating through their website at www.keeptahoeblue.org.

OPTIONS | Most successful summiteers will probably be content with the short but difficult climb of Thompson Peak.

WARM-UPS | A stop for baked goods at Hope Valley Café (14655 State Route 88) should reward you with some tasty treats for the drive or on the trail. If you want to sit and enjoy a meal, the café serves breakfast and lunch items from 7:00 AM to 5:00 PM. During the winter, you can take the chill off next to the roaring fire in the fireplace.

32 Grover Hot Springs State Park

Grover Hot Springs State Park is a winter oasis off the beaten track. Even though the park is open year-round, the area is relatively quiet in the winter months, beckoning snowshoers and Nordic skiers alike to its open meadows and serene forests. The nearly flat topography in the immediate vicinity around the park entrance provides easy snowshoeing opportunities for beginners and intermediates. More advanced users can venture into the more challenging terrain along Hot Springs and Charity Creeks.

LEVEL	Novice to intermediate
LENGTH	Varies, .5 mile to 3 miles, out and back to falls
TIME	1 hour to half day
ELEVATION	+425'–0'
DIFFICULTY	Easy to moderate
AVALANCHE RISK	Low
DOGS	On leash
FACILITIES	Campground, hot springs, ranger station, restrooms
MAP	SGS *Markleeville*
MANAGEMENT	Grover Hot Springs State Park at 530-694-2248, www.parks.ca.gov
HIGHLIGHTS	Creek, forest, meadows
LOWLIGHTS	Fee, variable snow conditions

TIP | With elevations at or below 6,000 feet, the snow conditions can be quite variable, depending on the weather. Call ahead to park headquarters for an update.

TRAILHEAD | 38°41.785'N, 119°50.090'W From the tiny community of Woodfords, drive south from the junction of State Route 88 and follow California State Route 89 for about 7 miles to the town of Markleeville. Turn right (west) in the center of town and follow Hot Springs Road for 3.5 miles to the entrance to Grover Hot Springs State Park. Unless you plan to use the hot springs pool, turn right at the entrance and park your vehicle in the day use lot near the picnic area, which doubles as the winter campground.

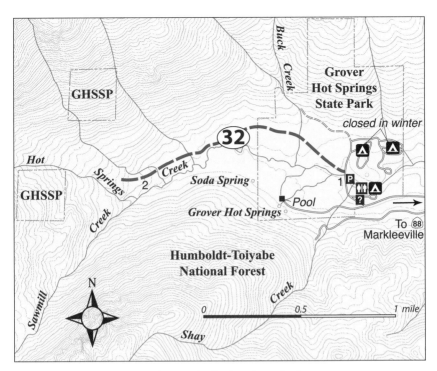

32. Grover Hot Springs State Park

ROUTE | [1] From either the day use or hot springs parking lots, head across the mostly open terrain of the meadows bordering Hot Springs Creek and head up the valley. Eventually the meadows are left behind, where the route enters a forest of western junipers, Jeffrey pines, and incense cedars. Beyond a small meadow [2], the canyon narrows and steepens, which is a good spot for some groups to turn around and head back to the trailhead [1]. More ambitious travelers can continue up the narrow and steep canyon of Hot Springs Creek to the waterfall, which is about one-quarter mile past the confluence of Sawmill Creek.

GROVER HOT SPRINGS The soothing waters in the pool at Grover Hot Springs State Park are the product of a subduction zone, at the collision point of tectonic plates, where one plate moves beneath the other. Intense pressure and friction from this collision combine to heat up rock to form superheated magma. In places where groundwater percolates through the earth's crust down to this magma, the heated water rises through faults and fractures and reaches the surface as a hot spring.

MILESTONES

1: Start at trailhead; 2: Small meadow; 1: Return to trailhead.

GO GREEN | Friends of Grover Hot Springs is a nonprofit organization dedicated to promoting relaxation and recreation, education, and preservation. You can learn more about their mission at www.visitgroverhotsprings.org.

OPTIONS | More experienced parties with good route-finding skills can continue up the canyon of Hot Springs Creek to Burnside Lake, or connect with Charity Valley Creek and head downstream to Charity Valley and Blue Lakes Road.

WARM-UPS | The hot springs pool remains open during the winter, although hours and days may vary. Usually the pool is open every day except Wednesdays and holidays. The fee to use the hot springs is not included in the park entrance fee and was $10 per person in 2017 ($5 for children). The park also transforms the picnic area into a campground ($25 per night) during the winter for tents and for trailers and motor homes under 18 feet long. For more information visit the park's website.

TRIP

33 | Hope Valley Overlook

A designated Nordic ski route follows the course of Forest Service Road 053 for 2.6 miles, followed by a 0.3-mile off-road jaunt to an overlook at the edge of a cliff, from where you'll have a fine view of Hope Valley and the surrounding terrain.

LEVEL	Novice to intermediate
LENGTH	5.8 miles, out and back
TIME	Three-quarter day
ELEVATION	+1,200'–275'
DIFFICULTY	Moderate
AVALANCHE RISK	Low
DOGS	OK
FACILITIES	Resort nearby
MAP	USGS *Freel Peak*
MANAGEMENT	Humboldt-Toiyabe National Forest at 775-882-2766, www.fs.usda.gov/htnf
HIGHLIGHTS	Forest, views
LOWLIGHTS	Parking, snowmobiles

TIP | Parking is extremely limited. An early arrival may increase your odds of acquiring a space. The Hope Valley SNO-PARK near the west end of the meadows has plenty of parking but is a very popular launching point for snow-mobiles, which have access to the meadows south of State Route 88.

TRAILHEAD | 38°46.478'N, 119°54.258'W From either Carson Valley in the east, or the Kirkwood area in the west, follow California State Route 88 to the vicinity of Hope Valley to the start of Forest Service Road 053, which is on the south side of the highway, 0.8 mile east of the junction of State Route 89 and directly west of Sorensen's Resort. Park your vehicle on the highway shoulder as space allows on either State Route 88 or 89.

ROUTE | [1] From State Route 88, begin on a winding climb along the course of the snow-covered road through a mixed forest of firs, pines, aspens, and an

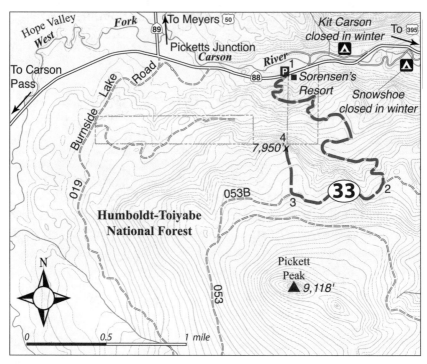

33. Hope Valley Overlook

occasional juniper. Blue diamond markers should help to keep you on route, but the course of the road is usually obvious. Follow a number of switchbacks up the hillside on a moderate to moderately steep ascent to where the grade eases for a while around the three-quarter-mile mark. After a brief respite, the climb resumes, leading to a spot where the trees part enough at one and three-quarter miles to allow a good view of Hope Valley and the surrounding peaks—a precursor to the much better views from the overlook. Soon enter back into forest cover and climb another one-quarter mile to a junction [2] with a road from Deep Canyon to the east.

Veer right (southwest) at the junction and make a westward traverse through a mixed forest of western white pines, red and white firs, lodgepole pines, and western junipers. At 2.6 miles you reach a point [3] directly north of Pickett Peak's summit, where you should turn north and head away from the road and begin the gradual descent toward point 7950.

Heading generally north, you follow the right-hand side of a bench toward the edge of some cliffs southeast of point 7950. After 0.3 mile, reach the edge of the overlook [4] with excellent, unobstructed views of Hope Valley and the terrain around Luther Pass, including snowy Waterhouse and Thompson Peaks. After fully admiring the views, retrace your steps to the trailhead [1].

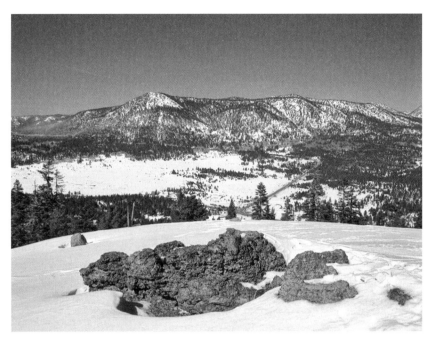

View from Hope Valley Overlook

MILESTONES
1: Start at trailhead; 2: Turn right at junction; 3: Turn right away from road; 4: Overlook; 1: Return to trailhead.

GO GREEN | Friends of Hope Valley is a nonprofit dedicated to the preservation and protection of Hope Valley and additional areas of eastern Alpine County. Learn more about the organization at www.friendsofhopevalley.org.

HOPE VALLEY Although the first non–Native Americans to visit Hope Valley were notables John C. Fremont and Kit Carson and members of their expedition in the winter of 1844, the area was named in 1848 by members of the disbanded Mormon Battalion on their return from the Mexican-American War. The lush grasses of Hope Valley were a staple for livestock for emigrant parties traveling the Carson River Route of the Emigrant Trail. Later, Carson Valley ranchers used the area as summer pasturage until the 1970s. A group of concerned Alpine County residents and supporters petitioned the state of California to purchase the undeveloped parcels of the valley, permanently protecting one of the largest subalpine meadows in the Sierra Nevada.

OPTIONS | An interesting trip extension would be a 0.6-mile, 1,050-foot climb of Pickett Peak for an even more outstanding view. Leave the road at Milestone 3 and head directly to the 9,118-foot summit.

The marked ski route continues on Road 053 to Burnside Lake Road. From there, you could head either northwest on the road to a pickup point at State Route 88 near the State Route 89 junction, or travel southeast to Burnside Lake and then take a more difficult and much longer route that follows the summertime hiking trail southeast to Charity Valley Creek and then east into Grover Hot Springs State Park.

WARM-UPS | Travelers on State Route 88 can dine on fresh-made cuisine at Sorensen's Resort, 0.9 mile east of the 88/89 junction. The charming café with a quaint mountain setting is open each day, serving breakfast from 7:30 AM to 11:00 AM, lunch from 11:00 AM to 4:00 PM, and dinner (reservations advised) from 5:00 PM to 8:30 PM. A variety of lodging is also available, from cozy bed-and-breakfast cottages to log cabins and rental homes. Visit their website at www.sorensensresort.com.

TRIP
34 | Hope Valley to Scotts Lake

The journey to Scotts Lake is a short, easy trip to a high mountain lake with spectacular views of the winter landscape east of Carson Pass.

LEVEL	Intermediate
LENGTH	3 miles, out and back
TIME	Half day
ELEVATION	+875'–0'
DIFFICULTY	Moderate
AVALANCHE RISK	Low
DOGS	OK
FACILITIES	None
MAP	USGS *Freel Peak*
MANAGEMENT	Humboldt-Toiyabe National Forest at 775-882-2766, www.fs.usda.gov/htnf
HIGHLIGHTS	Forest, lake, scenery
LOWLIGHT	Parking

TIP | You could follow the marked ski trail that follows the winding course of Forest Road 079 to Scotts Lake, but competent snowshoers can make a more direct approach by following the description below.

TRAILHEAD | 38°45.924'N, 119°56.404'W From either Carson Valley in the east, or the Kirkwood area in the west, follow California State Route 88 to the vicinity of Hope Valley and park your vehicle in a small plowed area on the west shoulder, 1.5 miles west of the Junction of State Route 89.

ROUTE | [1] From the edge of State Route 88, head directly toward a low saddle on the ridge just south of Waterhouse Peak, as Scotts Lake sits just below this saddle. Travel west across a flat and up the forested hillside on a moderate ascent. After a mile, the grade eases just before you reach the lake. Scotts Lake [2] offers a fine setting for admiring the splendid scenery, particularly the rugged north face of Stevens Peak. At the conclusion of your stay at the lake, retrace your steps to the trailhead [1].

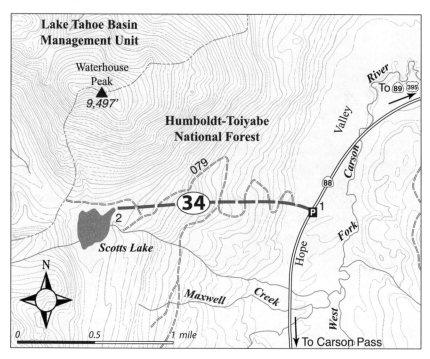

34. Hope Valley to Scotts Lake

MILESTONES
1: Start at trailhead; 2: Scotts Lake; 1: Return to trailhead.

GO GREEN | Friends of Hope Valley is a nonprofit dedicated to the preservation and protection of Hope Valley and additional areas of eastern Alpine County. Learn more about the organization at www.friendsofhopevalley.org.

OPTIONS | More ambitious, experienced snowshoers can accept the additional challenge of scaling nearby Waterhouse Peak. From Scotts Lake, climb steeply up the south ridge. About halfway up the mountain, the trees begin to thin and eventually all but disappear. Nearing what appears to be the top, you cross a small plateau to the base of the summit rocks, where a short, steep climb completes the ascent—the views are quite dramatic.

SUN CUPS Late in the season, as the Sierra snow begins the melt cycle, sun cups (also known as ablation hollows) can impede your progress over snow-covered slopes. They typically form on slopes of old snow during periods of prolonged sunshine, creating a field of similarly sized, bowl-shaped depressions.

As Scotts Lake is the same destination for Trip 28, two vehicles would allow you to create a 4.5-mile, point-to-point route between the Tahoe Rim Trailhead on State Route 89 and Hope Valley.

WARM-UPS | Travelers on State Route 88 can dine on fresh-made cuisine at Sorensen's Resort, 0.9 mile east of the 88/89 junction. The charming café with a quaint mountain setting is open each day, serving breakfast from 7:30 AM to 11:00 AM, lunch from 11:00 AM to 4:00 PM, and dinner (reservations advised) from 5:00 PM to 8:30 PM. A variety of lodging is also available, from cozy bed-and-breakfast cottages to log cabins and rental homes. Visit their website at www.sorensensresort.com.

35 Crater Lake

A short but steep ascent leads to a beautiful lake cradled in a dramatic cirque basin. While hundreds of weekend recreationists may be cavorting on the slopes around nearby Carson Pass, chances are you will have little company on this route, despite the minimal distance required to reach such a spectacular setting. Excellent views of the Hope Valley and Carson Pass areas en route complement the lake's stunning scenery.

LEVEL	Intermediate
LENGTH	3 miles, out and back
TIME	Half day
ELEVATION	+1,225'–0'
DIFFICULTY	Moderate
AVALANCHE RISK	Moderate
DOGS	OK
FACILITIES	None
MAP	USGS *Carson Pass*
MANAGEMENT	Humboldt-Toiyabe National Forest at 775-882-2766, www.fs.usda.gov/htnf
HIGHLIGHTS	Forest, lake, scenery
LOWLIGHT	Parking

TIP | Venturing close to the steep walls at the head of the canyon should only be done when snow conditions are stable. Check the current avalanche report at www.sierraavalanchecenter.org.

TRAILHEAD | 38°43.616'N, 119°57.248'W Follow California State Route 88 to an area westbound of Hope Valley and park your vehicle in a small plowed area on the west shoulder, 4.1 miles west of Picketts Junction with State Route 89 and 4.4 miles east of Carson Pass.

ROUTE | [1] Follow a moderately steep ascent just above the north bank of the creek draining Crater Lake on a route toward a low spot in the ridge above, located 0.85 mile southwest of Stevens Peak. Continue through a light mixed forest, composed of mainly lodgepole pines and ponderosa pines, with a

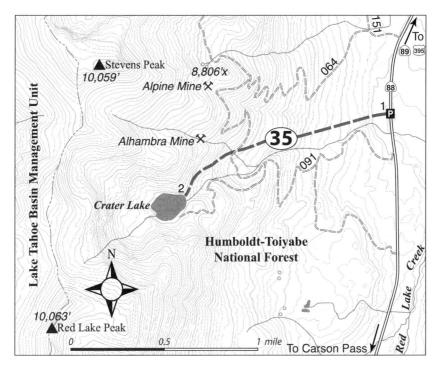

35. Crater Lake

lesser amount of white firs, and occasional incense cedars. Near the damp soils of the streambed, you'll also see some quaking aspens.

As you continue the ascent, the forest begins to thin, which allows for fine views of the areas around Hope Valley and Carson Pass. Nordic skiers tend to utilize a road system that zigzags up the slope on the opposite side of the drainage, but snowshoers can follow a more direct route up the moderately steep hillside. Nearing the head of the canyon, the grade steepens, necessitating an angling traverse to gentler slopes nearer the creek just below the

NORTHERN GOSHAWK (*Accipiter gentilis*) Year-round residents of Lake Tahoe, these raptors survive on rodents and birds. They are mostly gray in color with a bold white stripe above their piercing orange to red eyes. Females are larger than males by about 25 percent, and they are the primary nest sitters, keeping their eggs warm while the males hunt for prey. Goshawks are secretive birds that live primarily in thick forests, which makes a sighting by humans a rather rare occurrence. Development is the biggest threat to their continual presence in the Tahoe Basin.

rim of the lake's basin. Head upstream on a mellow grade for 500 feet before climbing a steeper slope to the rim, followed by a short drop to the east shore of Crater Lake [2].

Crater Lake is set in a spectacular amphitheater rimmed by steep rock walls midway between the towering summits of Stevens Peak to the north and Red Lake Peak to the south. From the lip of the basin, you have excellent views of the surrounding countryside. Retrace your steps to the trailhead [1].

MILESTONES

1: Start at trailhead; 2: Crater Lake; 1: Return to trailhead.

GO GREEN | Friends of Hope Valley is a nonprofit dedicated to the preservation and protection of Hope Valley and additional areas of eastern Alpine County. Learn more about the organization at www.friendsofhopevalley.org.

OPTIONS | For those with moderate mountaineering skills, 10,059-foot Stevens Peak is a reasonable goal.

WARM-UPS | Travelers on State Route 88 can dine on fresh-made cuisine at Sorensen's Resort, 0.9 mile east of the 88/89 junction. The charming café with a quaint mountain setting is open each day, serving breakfast from 7:30 AM to 11:00 AM, lunch from 11:00 AM to 4:00 PM, and dinner (reservations advised) from 5:00 PM to 8:30 PM. A variety of lodging is also available, from cozy bed-and-breakfast cottages to log cabins and rental homes. Visit their website at www.sorensensresort.com.

TRIP

36 | Red Lake Peak

Without mountaineering equipment and the technical expertise to use it, the true summit of Red Lake Peak may be beyond your grasp. However, a more easily accessible high point is only a stone's throw away and is only a few feet below the 10,063-foot top. Supreme views of Lake Tahoe and the mountainous terrain around Carson Pass are the chief rewards of the 1,500-foot ascent. The route is across mostly open slopes the entire way from the trailhead to the summit, which provides fantastic scenery but is also exposed to the elements.

LEVEL	Advanced
LENGTH	5 miles, out and back
TIME	Three-quarter day
ELEVATION	+1,500'–0'
DIFFICULTY	Strenuous
AVALANCHE RISK	Moderate to high
DOGS	Not recommended
FACILITIES	Vault toilets
MAPS	USGS *Caples Lake, Carson Pass*
MANAGEMENT	Eldorado National Forest at 209-295-4251, www.fs.usda.gov/eldorado
HIGHLIGHTS	Scenery, summit, views
LOWLIGHTS	Steep

TIP | Warning signs advise recreationists about the possibility of blasting for avalanche control along California State Route 88. The potential danger occurs on the steep slopes above the highway southeast of Red Lake Peak's summit. Avoid wandering off-route on the east side of the ridge.

TRAILHEAD | 38°41.800'N, 119°59.495'W The Meiss Meadow SNO-PARK (fee) is located off California State Route 88 on the north side of the road, 0.2 mile westbound of Carson Pass.

ROUTE | [1] From the parking lot, head west, generally contouring around the slopes of a lightly forested hillside. As you curve northwest into the drainage

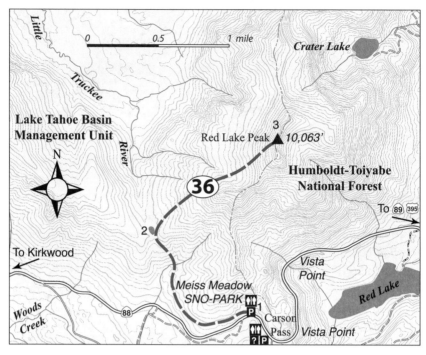

36. Red Lake Peak

of a minor tributary of Woods Creek, head for the obvious saddle ahead. Ascend open slopes, reaching the saddle [2] in a little over a mile from the SNO-PARK. The lack of trees allows for striking views to the south of Round Top and the surrounding peaks and ridges of the Carson Pass region.

Turning northeast from the saddle, you make an angling climb across moderately steep, wide-open slopes below Red Lake Peak. Follow a line of ascent that leads to the upper slopes of the mountain, curving beneath the first rock outcrop on the ridge above. Once beyond the outcrop the summit of Red Lake Peak pops into view, allowing you to follow a direct line toward the top. Head for the high point on the rounded ridge directly south of the group of rocks forming the true summit [3]. Difficult snow conditions may be encountered on the windswept slope near the top.

Similar to many crests in the Carson Pass area, the summit view from Red Lake Peak is quite dramatic, with Lake Tahoe glistening in the winter sun and surrounded by a ring of snowcapped peaks. The Crystal Range in Desolation Wilderness is particularly prominent. The immediate array of rugged peaks and canyons around Carson Pass composes one of the more dramatic landscapes in the greater Tahoe region. After completely enjoying the scenery, retrace your steps to the trailhead [1].

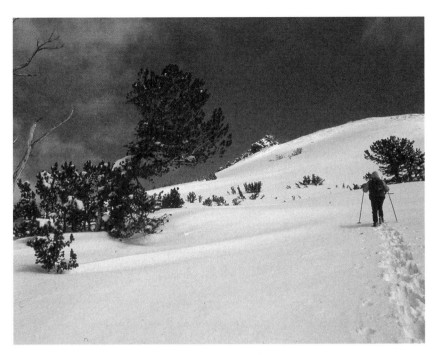

Climbing toward Red Lake Peak

MILESTONES

1: Start at trailhead; 2: Turn right at saddle; 3: Summit of Red Lake Peak; 1: Return to trailhead.

GO GREEN | You can support conservation of the greater Tahoe region by joining the Sierra Club, either through the Toiyabe (sierraclub.org/toiyabe) or Mother Lode (sierraclub.org/mother-lode) Chapters.

RED LAKE PEAK This 10,063-foot summit holds the distinction of being the vantage point from which the first Euro-Americans caught sight of Lake Tahoe. While on his second expedition to the American West, John C. Fremont, along with his chief cartographer, Charles Preuss, scaled Red Lake Peak on Valentine's Day of 1844, from where they saw the lake. Naming Carson Pass for guide Kit Carson, the expedition continued west down the American River valley to Sutter's Fort in present-day Sacramento. The most important discovery of Fremont's second expedition was that all the land in the Great Basin had no rivers connecting to the sea.

OPTIONS | The Upper Truckee River drainage offers plenty of backcountry for further explorations.

WARM-UPS | Westbound travelers on State Route 88 can grab lunch or dinner at the historic Kirkwood Inn and Saloon between 11:00 AM and 8:00 PM. The moderately priced establishment has served home-cooked meals for over 150 years and has a full bar. The inn is located on State Route 88, 0.4 mile west of Caples Lake. Visit the Kirkwood website at www.kirkwood.com/resort-services/resort-dining to view their menu. Call 209-258-7304 to confirm the current hours.

37 | Meiss and Showers Lakes

The journey to Meiss and Showers Lakes provides winter enthusiasts with a variety of impressive scenery. The first mile travels across wide-open slopes toward a saddle with superb views of the high mountains surrounding Carson Pass. Beyond the saddle, the expansive, gently sloping upper basin of the Upper Truckee River offers pleasant travel between tall ridges on the way to lovely Meiss Lake. The 7-mile round trip to Meiss Lake is a reasonable task, with the initial ascent to the saddle the only segment requiring much of a climb. Even though picturesque Showers Lake is just a little over a mile farther, a stiff ascent is needed to get there. With a low point at 8,300 feet, this route usually ensures an adequate snowpack throughout the winter season.

LEVEL	Intermediate to Meiss Lake; advanced to Showers Lake
LENGTH	7 miles, out and back to Meiss Lake; 10 miles, out and back to Showers Lake
TIME	Three-quarter day to Meiss Lake; full day to Showers Lake
ELEVATION	+400'–650' to Meiss Lake; +825–700' to Showers Lake
DIFFICULTY	Moderate to Meiss Lake; strenuous to Showers Lake
AVALANCHE RISK	Moderate
DOGS	OK
FACILITIES	Vault toilets
MAPS	USGS *Caples Lake*, *Carson Pass*
MANAGEMENT	Eldorado National Forest at 209-295-4251, www.fs.usda.gov/eldorado
HIGHLIGHTS	Lakes, scenery
LOWLIGHT	Steep (Showers Lake)

TIP | Depending on snow conditions, the trip all the way to Showers Lake may be a time-consuming endeavor. Since the area is at fairly high elevations with a long snow season, planning the trip later in the winter when daylight is longer might be wise.

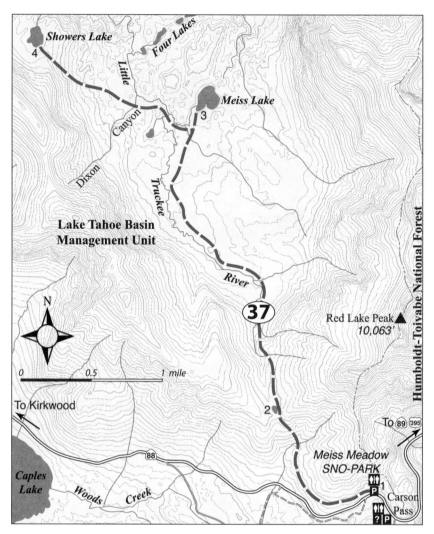

37. Meiss and Showers Lakes

TRAILHEAD | 38°41.800'N, 119°59.495'W The Meiss Meadow SNO-PARK (fee) is located off California State Route 88 on the north side of the road, 0.2 mile westbound of Carson Pass.

ROUTE | [1] The route to Meiss and Showers Lakes initially is the same as Trip 36 to Red Lake Peak. From the parking lot, head west, generally contouring around the slopes of a lightly forested hillside. As you curve northwest into the drainage of a minor tributary of Woods Creek, head for the obvious saddle ahead. Ascend open slopes, reaching the saddle [2] in a little over a mile from the SNO-PARK. The lack of trees allows for striking views to the south of Round Top and the surrounding peaks and ridges of the Carson Pass region.

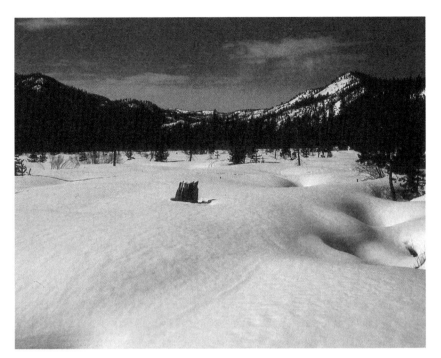

Meiss Lake

Leaving the saddle, which is the high point of the trip, a short, moderate descent leads north through a narrow drainage, where large cornices may appear along the western ridge crest. If the sight of these imposing cornices makes you queasy, pick a descent route well up the hillside on the east to avoid any possible avalanche run-outs. Beyond this potential hazard, you encounter more gentle terrain on the expansive floor of the Upper Truckee River canyon. The nearly level gradient of the upper basin provides for easy snowshoeing as you follow the general course of the frozen stream through widely scattered evergreens. The ridge to the west, which culminates in the broad summit of Little Round Top, provides a pleasantly scenic backdrop to the wide-open basin.

Even though the distance from the saddle to Meiss Lake is 2.5 miles, the gently descending grade of the upper basin provides the illusion of being much shorter. The pleasant scenery seemingly allows you to move quickly on the approach to the lake. Unless you're paying close attention, missing Meiss Lake is relatively easy, as the frozen body of water blends inconspicuously into the near-level and open floor of the basin. Reach Meiss Lake [3] at the northeast end of a large clearing, just below some low hills blanketed with a dense cover of trees. The delightful scenery of the basin should more than compensate for the lack of a discernible shoreline. If you're planning on going no farther than Meiss Lake, retrace your steps to the trailhead, remembering that the trip back to the saddle is uphill [1].

If you choose to go on to Showers Lake, head west across the open basin and over the course of the Upper Truckee River into more moderate forest cover. To reach the lake, leave the gentle terrain on the basin floor and begin a stiff climb up a tree-covered hillside, eventually roughly following the route of the summertime Pacific Crest Trail. Continue climbing until you crest the low ridge directly above the south shore, reaching picturesque Showers Lake [4] after a short drop, one and one-quarter miles from Meiss Lake and 5 miles from the SNO-PARK.

You can save some distance and time on the return trip by heading straight back along the course of the river, avoiding the slight detour to Meiss Lake. Where you rejoin your tracks, retrace your steps to the trailhead [1].

WHITE-TAILED PTARMIGAN (*Lagopus leucura*) The white-tailed ptarmigan is an introduced species in Lake Tahoe and the Sierra Nevada, and is the smallest of the birds in the grouse family. During summer, the bird's color is speckled grayish-brown with white underneath and on its tail and wings. However, in winter they turn totally white, which camouflages them quite well in the snow. Generally, these birds live exclusively in the higher elevations.

MILESTONES

1: Start at trailhead; 2: Saddle; 3: Meiss Lake; 4: Showers Lake; 1: Return to trailhead.

GO GREEN | Snowlands Network is a fine organization dedicated to protecting winter human-powered recreation across public lands. Consult their website at www.snowlands.org.

OPTIONS | Most snowshoers will be satisfied with the trip to either Meiss or Showers Lakes as more than enough activity for one day.

WARM-UPS | Westbound travelers on State Route 88 can grab lunch or dinner at the historic Kirkwood Inn and Saloon between 11:00 AM and 8:00 PM. The moderately priced establishment has served home-cooked meals for over 150 years and has a full bar. The inn is located on State Route 88, 0.4 mile west of Caples Lake. Visit the Kirkwood website at www.kirkwood.com/resort -services/resort-dining to view their menu. Call 209-258-7304 to confirm the current hours.

Little Round Top

This little-known trip to the summit of Little Round Top offers nearly continuous, awe-inspiring views of some beautiful scenery near and far. Beyond the first mile, the route follows an exposed ridge for another 4 miles, where snowshoers are treated to some of the best scenery in the greater Tahoe area. Even those short on time and unable to complete the full out-and-back trip could turn around at any point along the ridge and still be more than satisfied with the views.

This trip is a good choice for novices, as the ridge route requires only minimal route finding—simply gain the ridge and follow it to the top—and the terrain is not particularly steep for any great length. However, the distance involved does require a fair amount of physical endurance and stamina.

LEVEL	Intermediate
LENGTH	10.5 miles, out and back
TIME	Full day
ELEVATION	+1,600'–500'
DIFFICULTY	Strenuous
AVALANCHE RISK	Low to moderate
DOGS	OK
FACILITIES	Vault toilets
MAPS	USGS *Caples Lake, Carson Pass*
MANAGEMENT	Eldorado National Forest at 209-295-4251, www.fs.usda.gov/eldorado
HIGHLIGHTS	Scenery, summit, views
LOWLIGHT	Cornices

TIP | Avoid the usually corniced right-hand side of the ridge leading toward Little Round Top. Almost the entire route is near or above 9,000 feet and along a treeless, exposed ridge where stiff winds are not uncommon. Plan on visiting when winds are forecast to be light.

TRAILHEAD | 38°41.800'N, 119°59.495'W The Meiss Meadow SNO-PARK (fee) is located off California State Route 88 on the north side of the road, 0.2 mile westbound of Carson Pass.

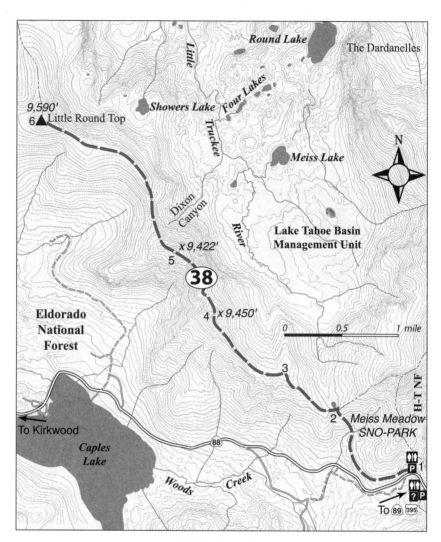

38. Little Round Top

ROUTE | [1] The route to Little Round Top initially is the same as Trip 36 to Red Lake Peak and Trip 37 to Meiss and Showers Lakes. From the parking lot, head west, generally contouring around the slopes of a lightly forested hillside. As you curve northwest into the drainage of a minor tributary of Woods Creek, head for the obvious saddle ahead. The lack of trees allows for striking views to the south of Round Top and the surrounding peaks and ridges of the Carson Pass region. Just before the saddle **[2]**, bear left and ascend a moderately steep slope a short way to gain the top of the ridge.

Follow the ridge crest over gentle terrain until reaching the base of the first high point, where the grade increases to moderate. Climb to the top of this high point **[3]**, 1.8 miles from the trailhead, from where you have fine

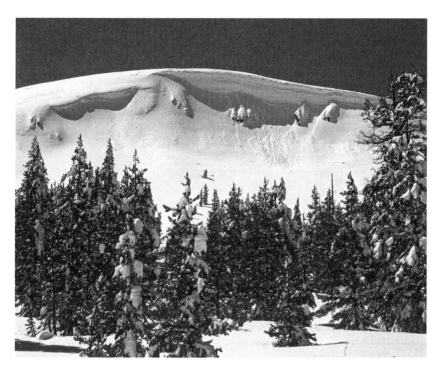
A massive cornice on Little Round Top

views south to Round Top Peak and north to Lake Tahoe. If you're looking for a shorter trip, this spot would make a good turnaround point.

As you descend, the ridge bends slightly west, providing a chilling view of some nasty-looking cornices that frequently form on the east side of the ridge ahead. Where the ridge narrows and curves back to the north, make a gently ascending traverse over to the base of a significant peak and then climb steeper slopes to the 9,450-foot top [4], 2.6 miles from the trailhead. As expected, the view from this aerie is magnificent, including the meadows bordering the Upper Truckee River in the valley below to the northwest, as well as the snowy peaks around the Carson Pass and Lake Tahoe areas.

CORNICES Average and above-average winters produce some nasty-looking cornices on Little Round Top. From the Italian word for ledge, cornices are overhanging masses of snow deposited by the wind. Potentially dangerous, a cornice can break off the side of a ridge under its own weight or can be triggered by the weight of unsuspecting humans traveling too close to the edge. When cornices do break, they can produce significant avalanches, creating a potential hazard for anyone beneath them.

A moderate, one-quarter-mile descent leads away from the high point and down to a saddle. From there, follow the ridge north-northwest up gentle slopes to the next high point. A short descent leads to another saddle, after which you ascend once again, reaching Peak 9422 [5] at 3.3 miles from the trailhead.

A drop of a half mile brings you to the start of the final, lengthy climb along the ridge to the top of Little Round Top. Initially, the route ascends over moderate slopes to Point 9325, beyond which the terrain mellows considerably, as the ridge sweeps around to the west. For the next three-quarter mile, the grade is quite easy, followed by a short, moderate climb to the summit of Little Round Top [6].

Even more spectacular views greet you at the top, where an unobstructed vista sweeps across a vast area of the northern Sierra, extending from north Tahoe peaks to the mountains around Sonora Pass. The more immediate topography is both dramatic and striking in its majesty, especially the airy summits found in both Desolation and Mokelumne Wilderness Areas. The return trip to the trailhead [1] promises another 5 miles of great views and wonderful scenery.

MILESTONES

1: Start at Meiss Meadows SNO-PARK; 2: Saddle; 3: High point; 4: Peak 9,450; 5: Peak 9,422; 6: Little Round Top; 1: Return to trailhead.

GO GREEN | You can support conservation of the greater Tahoe region by joining the Sierra Club, either through the Toiyabe (sierraclub.org/toiyabe) or Mother Lode (sierraclub.org/mother-lode) Chapters.

OPTIONS | Most winter users will be content to go no farther than the summit of Little Round Top.

WARM-UPS | Westbound travelers on State Route 88 can grab lunch or dinner at the historic Kirkwood Inn and Saloon between 11:00 AM and 8:00 PM. The moderately priced establishment has served home-cooked meals for over 150 years and has a full bar. The inn is located on State Route 88, 0.4 mile west of Caples Lake. Visit the Kirkwood website at www.kirkwood.com/resort -services/resort-dining to view their menu. Call 209-258-7304 to confirm the current hours.

Winnemucca
and Round Top Lakes

The Carson Pass region boasts of some of the most inspiring terrain in the greater Lake Tahoe area. Combined with a high-elevation start from the 8,652-foot-high pass that usually ensures good snow conditions and straightforward access from a SNO-PARK, the spectacular scenery draws a high number of winter recreationists throughout the season. A ban on snowmobiles certainly doesn't hurt the area's popularity among the human-powered crowd, either. The route described here leads winter users to two of the prettiest lakes, backdropped by an amphitheater of rugged peaks that include the smooth contour of Elephants Back and the rugged rock of Round Top, The Sisters, and Black Butte.

LEVEL	Intermediate
LENGTH	6.5 miles, loop
TIME	Full day
ELEVATION	+1,500'–1,500'
DIFFICULTY	Moderate
AVALANCHE RISK	Moderate
DOGS	OK
FACILITIES	Vault toilets
MAPS	USGS *Caples Lake*, *Carson Pass*
MANAGEMENT	Eldorado National Forest at 209-295-4251, www.fs.usda.gov/eldorado
HIGHLIGHTS	Forest, lake, scenery
LOWLIGHT	Popular

TIP | Get an early start on sunny weekends, as the parking lot tends to fill up quickly.

TRAILHEAD | 38°41.712'N, 119°59.372'W The Carson Pass SNO-PARK (fee) is located on California State Route 88 on the south side of the road at Carson Pass.

ROUTE | [1] Head south from the parking area into moderate forest cover, skirting the west side of the ridge forming the divide running generally southeast.

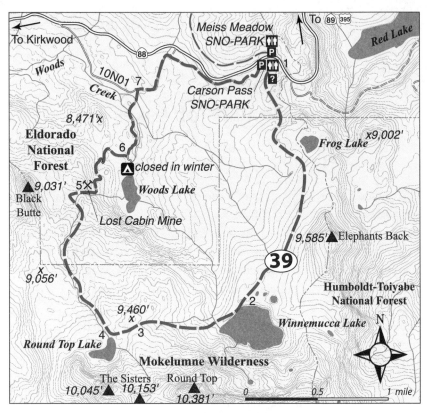

39. Winnemucca and Round Top Lakes

After one-quarter mile of gently rising terrain, you start climbing more moderately, breaking out into more open terrain after about another one-quarter mile. Pass to the west of Frog Lake and continue the ascent across the open, west slopes of Elephants Back. Wind-packed snow in this vicinity may produce less than ideal snow conditions along the traverse, but they should improve on the way to the lake. Reach the north shore of Winnemucca Lake [2] at 1.8 miles from the trailhead, where scattered whitebark pines provide little shelter from the prevailing winds. The towering north face of 10,381-foot Round Top looms above the 8,980-foot lake. If you're pressed for time, Winnemucca Lake is a good turnaround point for a half-day excursion.

Leave the shore of Winnemucca Lake and head west up the drainage of a tributary stream on a three-quarter-mile climb to a 9,460-foot saddle on the northwest ridge of Round Top separating the basins of Winnemucca and Round Top Lakes. From the saddle [3], make a short descent to the north shore of picturesque Round Top Lake [4].

To continue the circuit, follow the outlet northwest for about a half mile and then north-northeast for another half mile or so to a flat just to the east

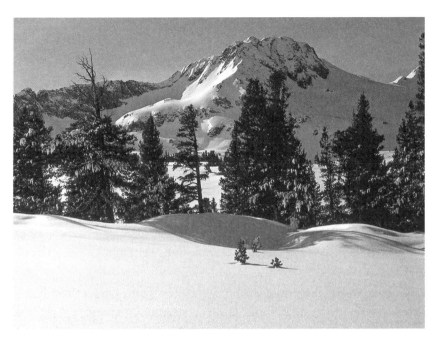

Winnemucca Lake backdropped by Round Top

of Black Butte. From the south side of the flat, head east to the edge and drop downslope for a short distance to Lost Cabin Mine [5], where you can pick up the course of the narrow mine road heading north and then east toward the more discernible Woods Lake Road [6]. Follow Woods Lake Road for half a mile to a junction [7] on the far side of Woods Creek.

Turn right (east) and follow this section of road for a little over a mile to State Route 88, across from the entrance to the Meiss Meadow SNO-PARK on the opposite shoulder. From there, follow the course of the highway uphill back to your vehicle at the Carson Pass SNO-PARK [1].

KIT CARSON Christopher Houston Carson (1809–1868) grew up in Missouri but left at the age of sixteen to become a mountain man and trapper in the American West. In the 1840s, he was hired as a guide for John C. Fremont's expedition to California, Oregon, and the Great Basin. He later fought in the Mexican-American War under Fremont and then led a regiment of mostly Hispanic volunteers from New Mexico in the Civil War. His exploits as a mountain man became legend and were exaggerated in dime novels. Numerous landmarks now bear his name, including Carson Pass, Carson City, Carson Range, Carson Spur, and Carson Canyon.

1: Start at Carson Pass trailhead; 2: Winnemucca Lake; 3: Saddle; 4: Round Top Lake; 5: Lost Cabin Mine; 6: Turn left at Woods Lake Road; 7: Turn right at junction; 1: Return to Carson Pass trailhead.

GO GREEN | You can learn about the work of the Sierra Nevada Alliance to protect Sierra waterways, open space, wildlife habitat, working landscapes, and scenic views by visiting their website at www.sierranevadaalliance.com.

OPTIONS | Some experienced mountaineers attempt winter ascents of Round Top. From Round Top Lake, head southeast up a gully toward the saddle between The Sisters and Round Top. Before gaining the saddle, veer left toward a notch in the ridge above and then follow the ridge toward a false summit. Depending on the conditions, the slightly lower false summit may end up as the goal, as the true summit requires some difficult climbing with a fair bit of exposure.

WARM-UPS | Westbound travelers on State Route 88 can grab lunch or dinner at the historic Kirkwood Inn and Saloon between 11:00 AM and 8:00 PM. The moderately priced establishment has served home-cooked meals for over 150 years and has a full bar. The inn is located on State Route 88, 0.4 mile west of Caples Lake. Visit the Kirkwood website at www.kirkwood.com/resort -services/resort-dining to view their menu. Call 209-258-7304 to confirm the current hours.

TRIP
40 Echo Lakes

Beginning snowshoers will love this journey, which follows a nearly flat, well-marked road to the wide-open expanse of Lower and Upper Echo Lakes. More experienced travelers may recognize this route as the gateway into the dramatic scenery within Desolation Wilderness, offering tantalizing temptations for a lengthy day trip or perhaps a multiday outing. The open terrain of the frozen lakes allows users to tailor the length of trips to the specific skills and conditioning of their group. A round trip of 2 miles leads to the shore of Lower Echo Lake and back, while the full journey to Upper Echo Lake lengthens the round-trip journey to 6.5 miles. The gentle terrain, lack of route finding, and flexibility of choosing the distance are attributes that both novices and more experienced snowshoers should appreciate.

The scenery is fantastic, with sheer rock cliffs and tall ridges rising sharply above the shoreline and providing a fine backdrop to the smoothly frozen surface of the lakes. Talking Mountain climbs nearly 1,500 feet above the lower lake, and, on the opposite side of the basin, Echo Peak soars to a similar height above the upper lake.

The ease of approach coupled with the beautiful surroundings makes the trip to Echo Lakes quite popular. Expect plenty of company if you plan to be here on a sunny weekend day. Fortunately for the human-powered crowd, snowmobiles are only allowed on the road for government business and access to private homes.

LEVEL Novice to intermediate
LENGTH Varies, 2 to 6.5 miles, out and back
TIME 2 hours to three-quarter day
ELEVATION Negligible
DIFFICULTY Easy to moderate
AVALANCHE RISK Low to moderate
DOGS OK
FACILITIES Port-a-potty
MAP USGS *Echo Lake*

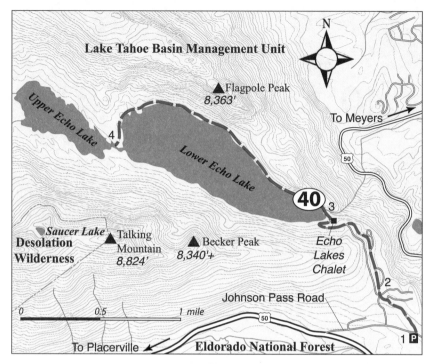

40. Echo Lakes

MANAGEMENT Lake Tahoe Basin Management Unit at 530-543-2600,
www.fs.usda.gov/ltbmu

HIGHLIGHTS Lake, scenery

LOWLIGHT Popular

TIP | Arrive early on sunny weekends to secure a parking spot.

TRAILHEAD | 38°49.415'N, 120°02.031'W From U.S. 50, find the signed turnoff for the Echo Lakes SNO-PARK, 1 mile westbound of Echo Summit. Follow the narrow, plowed Johnson Pass Road for a half mile to a right-hand turn into the parking area.

ROUTE | [1] Find the start of the trail to Echo Lakes opposite the entrance into the SNO-PARK and follow the snow-covered Echo Lakes Road (FS 11N05) northbound on a usually packed trail (popular with recreationists, Cal-Trans also occasionally runs snow-cats along the road to access the steep slopes above U.S. 50 for avalanche control). Continue along the road for nearly half a mile to a junction [2] with a road on the right to Berkeley Muni Camp.

Veer left at the junction to remain on Echo Lakes Road and pass by a number of summer homes on a gently rising grade toward Lower Echo Lake. Just prior to the lake, the road starts to descend, makes a hairpin turn, and soon reaches the shoreline [3], about 1 mile from the SNO-PARK.

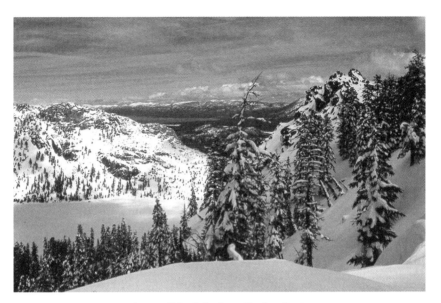
Lower Echo Lake from Becker Peak

Once at Lower Echo Lake, you can tailor your trip to suit the desires of your group, with the open and flat terrain well suited for explorations of varying lengths. In all but the mildest of winters, the lake freezes deep enough to allow unrestricted travel over the surface. However, check the current conditions and only travel across the lake with extreme caution and at your own risk. In particular, avoid the areas near the inlet and outlet, as the slightly moving water tends to thaw before the rest of the lake. Stay off the surface on both lakes when spring temperatures begin to rise. The safest plan is to stick to the lakeshore and avoid the lake altogether. If desired, continue all the way to Upper Echo Lake [4].

Please respect the private property in the area by traveling away from the summer homes and cabins surrounding the lakes. Otherwise, enjoy the area at your own pace, traveling only as far as you choose. When the time comes, return to the SNO-PARK [1].

TROUT IN THE WINTER Echo Lakes are home to several species of fish, including Kokanee salmon; Lahontan cutthroat, rainbow, and brook trout. During the winter, when the water temperature drops, the metabolism of these cold-blooded creatures slows considerably. However, trout can be more active than a lot of other species that prefer deeper waters. Trout oftentimes reside in a band just three to six inches below the ice.

1: Start at trailhead; 2: Left at junction; 3: Lower Echo Lake; 4: Upper Echo Lake; 1: Return to trailhead.

GO GREEN | You can support conservation of the greater Tahoe region by joining the Sierra Club, either through the Toiyabe (sierraclub.org/toiyabe) or Mother Lode (sierraclub.org/mother-lode) Chapters.

OPTIONS | Those who enjoy winter camping can extend their journey into Desolation Wilderness beyond Upper Echo Lake. Just as in the warmer months, a wilderness permit is required for all overnight stays, available from ranger stations of the Lake Tahoe Basin Management Unit or Eldorado National Forest.

WARM-UPS | In the shadow of famed Lover's Leap, the historic Strawberry Lodge, once a stop on the Pony Express, has been serving travelers since 1858. The wood-paneled dining room is a fine setting for enjoying good, hearty food before or after a spin in the backcountry. During winter, weekday diners can select from the breakfast menu from 7:30 AM to 12 noon, or the lunch menu from 11:00 AM to 8:30 PM. The dinner menu is available from Friday to Sunday nights between 5:00 PM and 8:30 PM. The lodge also has numerous guest rooms and a streamside cabin for overnight stays. Find Strawberry Lodge at 17150 Highway 50, approximately 9 miles east of Kyburz and 9 miles west of Echo Summit. For more information, visit their website at www.strawberrylodge.com or call 530-659-7200.

Becker Peak

A reasonably short trip without a tremendous amount of elevation gain leads to a supreme view of the South Lake Tahoe region. You probably won't be alone on the first part of the journey, as the route follows the popular route to Echo Lakes, but once you leave the road behind and head toward Becker Peak, the masses are usually left behind. Away from a marked trail, the route finding is not particularly difficult—simply follow a distinct ridge to the summit. Depending on snow conditions, the final slope below the top may require some extra skill to negotiate. The ascent of Becker Peak is definitely a trip where a great reward requires a correspondingly limited amount of effort.

LEVEL	Intermediate to advanced
LENGTH	3.4 miles, out and back
TIME	Half day
ELEVATION	+950'–0'
DIFFICULTY	Moderate
AVALANCHE RISK	Moderate
DOGS	OK
FACILITIES	Port-a-potty
MAP	USGS *Echo Lake*
MANAGEMENT	Lake Tahoe Basin Management Unit at 530-543-2600, www.fs.usda.gov/ltbmu
HIGHLIGHTS	Summit, views
LOWLIGHT	Snow conditions

TIP | Depending on conditions, carrying an ice axe and crampons might be helpful on the upper part of the climb.

TRAILHEAD | 38°49.415'N, 120°02.031'W From U.S. 50, find the signed turnoff for the Echo Lakes SNO-PARK, 1 mile westbound of Echo Summit. Follow the narrow, plowed Johnson Pass Road for half a mile to a right-hand turn into the parking area.

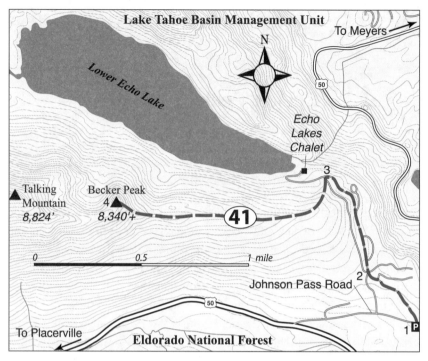

41. Becker Peak

ROUTE | [1] The initial part of the journey from the SNO-PARK is the same as in Trip 41 to Echo Lakes. Find the start of the trail to Echo Lakes opposite the entrance into the SNO-PARK and follow the snow-covered Echo Lakes Road (FS 11N05) northbound on a usually packed trail (popular with winter users, Cal-Trans also occasionally runs snow-cats along the road to access the steep slopes above U.S. 50 for avalanche control). Continue along the road for nearly half a mile to a junction [2] with a road on the right to Berkeley Muni Camp.

Veer left at the junction to remain on Echo Lakes Road and pass by a number of summer homes on a gently rising grade toward Lower Echo Lake. Instead of continuing all the way to the lake, leave the road at the high point near a curve, about 0.8 mile from the SNO-PARK [3]. Here, both Lake Tahoe and Becker Peak come into view.

Turn left from the road and head generally west on a moderately steep climb across a lightly forested hillside to gain the top of a ridge. Where the grade eases, you have filtered views of Lake Tahoe in the distance and Lower Echo Lake directly below. Follow the ridge on a gentle ascent for a mile of pleasant snowshoeing through a light cover of firs and pines. Toward the end of the ridge, just before Becker Peak, pass a small pinnacle on the left, traversing across a high-angle slope. Past this minor obstacle, reach the final,

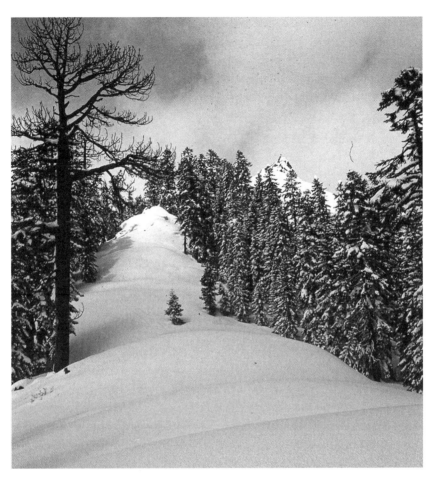
The ridge leading to Becker Peak

steep slope below the summit. The last 150 feet of the ascent will likely be the most difficult part of the route, as the steep angle of the slope combined with less than ideal snow conditions may require some careful maneuvering. The summit is composed of a conglomeration of large, usually bare rocks, which can produce some tricky footing when coated with a thin covering of snow or ice. You can elect to pick your way around the rocks, or simply drop your snowshoes for the last pitch.

BECKER PEAK The mountain was named for a local resident, John S. Becker, who homesteaded some land near Lower Echo Lake for a cattle ranch. In 1886, he built a cabin that was later expanded. He also ran a successful saloon according to the *Tahoe Tattler*.

However you choose to gain the summit [4], the view from Becker Peak is sublime, with Echo Lakes providing a beautiful sight at the gateway into the dramatic mountain scenery of Desolation Wilderness. The south part of Lake Tahoe appears farther on and the trio of Freel Peak, Jobs Sister, and Jobs Peak lies to the east. When the time comes, retrace your steps to the trailhead [1].

MILESTONES

1: Start at trailhead; 2: Left at junction; 3: Turn left at curve; 4: Becker Peak; 1: Return to trailhead.

GO GREEN | You can assist the Eldorado National Forest by volunteering for a variety of projects. Consult their website at www. fs.usda.gov/main/Eldorado /workingtogether/volunteering.

OPTIONS | You can extend the trip by following the ridge from Becker Peak another half mile to an even better view from Talking Mountain. The ascent, although steeper than the climb to Becker Peak, is straightforward and not particularly difficult, with a couple of caveats. First, avoid the cornices along the north side of the ridge. Second, around the midpoint of the climb between Becker and Talking Mountain, you must pass a large rock outcropping. This area of rock presents a thin covering of snow, which makes for less than ideal purchase for your snowshoes. In addition, a preponderance of brush carpets the hillsides between the rocks, which may also make the slopes difficult to negotiate during periods of limited snowfall. Combine these elements with a certain amount of exposure down the steep slopes to the south and this extension can be recommended only for experienced mountain travelers.

WARM-UPS | In the shadow of famed Lover's Leap, the historic Strawberry Lodge, once a stop on the Pony Express, has been serving travelers since 1858. The wood-paneled dining room is a fine setting for enjoying good, hearty food before or after a spin in the backcountry. During winter, weekday diners can select from the breakfast menu from 7:30 AM to 12 noon, or the lunch menu from 11 AM to 8:30 PM. The dinner menu is available from Friday to Sunday nights between 5:00 PM and 8:30 PM. The lodge also has numerous guest rooms and a streamside cabin for overnight stays. Find Strawberry Lodge at 17150 Highway 50, approximately 9 miles east of Kyburz and 9 miles west of Echo Summit. For more information, visit their website at www.strawberry lodge.com or call 530-659-7200.

42 | Ralston Peak

A trip to the top of Ralston Peak will bless visitors with incredible vistas in all directions. From the ridge crest along the way, the view down into Pyramid Creek Canyon is equally impressive. The price for such beautiful scenery is a moderately steep, continuous, 2.5-mile climb that gains 2,700 vertical feet. However, physically fit intermediate snowshoers should have no other problems along the way, as the terrain is straightforward. Due to limited parking near the trailhead, the area is very lightly used in the winter.

LEVEL	Intermediate to advanced
LENGTH	5 miles, out and back
TIME	Full day
ELEVATION	+2,800'–100'
DIFFICULTY	Strenuous
AVALANCHE RISK	Moderate
DOGS	OK
FACILITIES	None
MAP	USGS *Echo Lake*
MANAGEMENT	Lake Tahoe Basin Management Unit at 530-543-2600, www.fs.usda.gov/ltbmu
HIGHLIGHTS	Summit, views
LOWLIGHTS	Parking, steep

TIP | As parking may be extremely limited, this is probably not the best trip for a group outing.

TRAILHEAD | 38°48.204'N, 120°07.076'W Finding a place to park your vehicle may likely be the most difficult part of this trip. Along U.S. 50, 4.8 miles westbound of Echo Summit, find a small plowed area on the shoulder barely big enough for four to five vehicles. This space is near Camp Sacramento, at the beginning of a paved access road.

ROUTE | [1] Carefully cross Highway 50 and begin climbing up the hillside above the westbound lanes. Pass through a moderate cover of mixed forest, heading for the ridgeline to the east of Pyramid Creek's precipitous canyon.

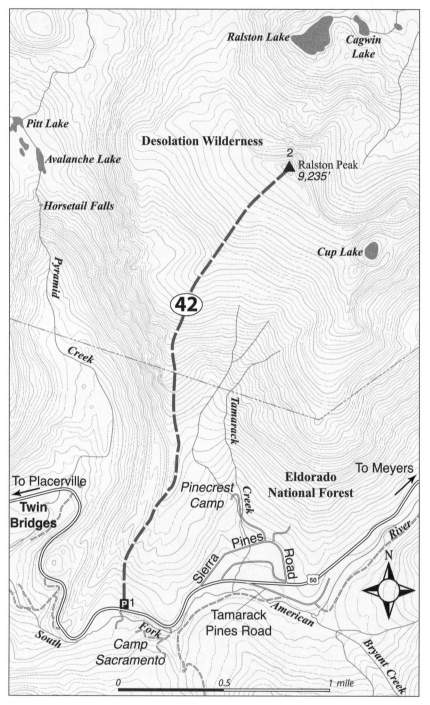

42. Ralston Peak

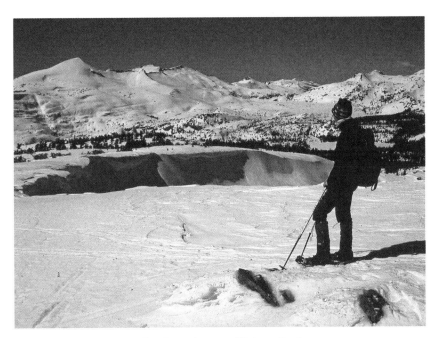

View from the top of Ralston Peak

Where you gain the crest are staggering views down into this declivity and of Horsetail Falls spilling down the headwall. The views improve even farther up the ridge, where Pyramid Peak and Mount Price rise above the deep gorge.

Continue the ascent along the ridge, dropping down from the crest on occasion to pass some steep projections. Ralston Peak is not an impressive-looking mountain, lacking the alpine flair of its neighbors across the canyon to the west. However, the view *from* the top will be more than compensation for the pedestrian view *of* the top.

About one and three-quarter miles into the journey, bend northeast and head directly for the summit of Ralston Peak. The trees begin to thin as you gain elevation—ultimately the only conifers that remain are some weather-beaten and twisted whitebark pines. Finally reach the broad summit at 2.5 miles from Highway 50 [2].

As promised, the view from the top is magnificent, with Pyramid Peak and other summits in Desolation Wilderness the dominant attraction immediately to the west. Directly below lie the frozen surfaces of Ralston, Cagwin, and Tamarack Lakes, and to the east the much larger Echo Lakes. Across Lake Tahoe farther east is Freel Peak, highest summit in the basin, flanked by Jobs Peak and Jobs Sister. Between Echo Peak and Mount Tallac, Lake Tahoe sweeps away to the north. To the south are Lovers Leap directly below and the mountains around Carson Pass farther out.

William Chapman Ralston Raised in Ohio, William Chapman Ralston (1826–1875), worked on Mississippi riverboats before making his way west to California as a captain aboard a ship bringing Central American workers to the Comstock Lode. He teamed with Darius Ogden Mills to open the Bank of California in San Francisco and was a major player in the development of the city's financial district. He lived large through numerous successes and failures while maintaining a sense of modesty usually missing in men of means. He drowned while swimming in San Francisco Bay.

MILESTONES

1: Start at trailhead; 2: Summit of Mount Ralston; 1: Return to trailhead.

GO GREEN | You can support conservation of the greater Tahoe region by joining the Sierra Club, either through the Toiyabe (sierraclub.org/toiyabe) or Mother Lode (sierraclub.org/mother-lode) Chapters.

OPTIONS | An early start, an ample supply of extra energy, and arrangements for a car shuttle would enable you to consider an exciting 10-mile loop trip. From the summit of Ralston Peak, head northwest and then north to Haypress Meadows (avoiding the steep terrain directly north of the summit). From the meadows, head down the drainage of Echo Creek, generally following the route of the Pacific Crest Trail, to Upper and Lower Echo Lakes and then down the snow-covered Echo Lakes Road to the Echo Summit SNO-PARK.

WARM-UPS | In the shadow of famed Lover's Leap, the historic Strawberry Lodge, once a stop on the Pony Express, has been serving travelers since 1858. The wood-paneled dining room is a fine setting for enjoying good, hearty food before or after a spin in the backcountry. During winter, weekday diners can select from the breakfast menu from 7:30 AM to 12 noon, or the lunch menu from 11:00 AM to 8:30 PM. The dinner menu is available from Friday to Sunday nights between 5:00 PM and 8:30 PM. The lodge also has numerous guest rooms and a streamside cabin for overnight stays. Find Strawberry Lodge at 17150 Highway 50, approximately 9 miles east of Kyburz and 9 miles west of Echo Summit. For more information, visit their website at www.strawberry lodge.com or call 530-659-7200.

TRIP 43 | Angora Lookout and Angora Lakes

Throngs of summer visitors to the Fallen Leaf Lake area are permitted to drive their vehicles all the way to Angora Lookout for a superb view, and most of the distance beyond to lower Angora Lake for a day of fishing, boating, swimming, or sunbathing. Although snowmobilers are afforded the same freedom of access in the winter, the lookout and lakes see far fewer visitors. The view from the lookout is still exceptional and the lakes take on a much more peaceful ambiance when frozen and snow blankets the shoreline.

The route to Angora Lookout follows an unbending, snow-covered road all the way to the top, requiring little in the way of route-finding ability. The journey beyond the lookout to Angora Lakes is fairly straightforward as well, but does necessitate a bit more navigational skill.

LEVEL	Intermediate
LENGTH	4 miles, out and back to Lookout; 7 miles, out and back to Upper Angora Lake
TIME	Half day to Lookout; full day to lakes
ELEVATION	+650'–50' to lookout; +875'–125' to Upper Angora Lake
DIFFICULTY	Moderate
AVALANCHE RISK	Moderate
DOGS	OK
FACILITIES	None
MAPS	USGS *Echo Lake, Emerald Bay*
MANAGEMENT	Lake Tahoe Basin Management Unit at 530-543-2600, www.fs.usda.gov/ltbmu
HIGHLIGHTS	Lakes, views
LOWLIGHTS	Recent forest fire, limited parking, snowmobiles

TIP | Angora Lookout is an excellent spot from which to observe the geology of the region, including numerous moraines left by retreating glaciers, as well as some cirque basins. Pack along a small-scale map to help identify the numerous landmarks visible from the lookout.

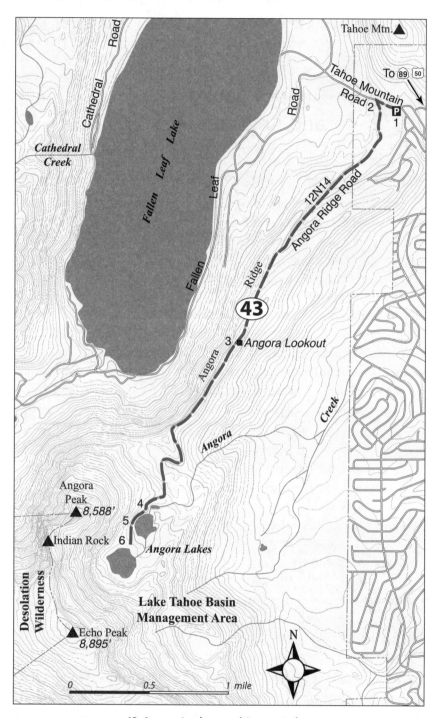

43. Angora Lookout and Angora Lakes

TRAILHEAD | 38°54.189′N, 120°02.168′W From the Y in South Lake Tahoe, where Highways 50 and 89 meet, head southwest on Lake Tahoe Boulevard for 2.4 miles and turn right onto Tahoe Mountain Road. After a mile, turn right onto Glenmore Way and then immediately left onto Dundee Circle. Follow Dundee Circle to an intersection with Tahoe Mountain Road again, turn left, and park your vehicle nearby as space allows.

ROUTE | [1] From where you parked your vehicle, descend along Tahoe Mountain Road for 0.1 mile to the beginning of Angora Ridge Road (FS 12N14) [2]. Turn left and head south, passing a meadow lined with quaking aspens. Beyond the meadow, continue ahead, following the course of the road through a mixed forest of pines, firs, and cedars. After half a mile, the road begins to climb gradually steeper and the steady ascent eventually leads toward the crest of Angora Ridge, where partial views tease the visitor with expectations of even better vistas to come. Nearing the top, utility lines crossing above the road hint at the location of the Angora Lookout [3], around 2 miles from the trailhead.

The view from the lookout is spectacular. Fallen Leaf Lake is not quite 1,000 feet directly below, seemingly a stone's throw away. The impressive east face of dark, 9,735-foot Mount Tallac is a looming hulk above the far side of the lake. To the north is a slice of Lake Tahoe, glistening in the low-angled rays of the winter sun. The snowcapped summit of Mount Ralston dominates a ridge of peaks standing guard over the southern boundary of Desolation Wilderness. Freel Peak, highest mountain in the Tahoe Basin, appears in the distance to the southwest. If you're only going as far as the lookout, retrace your steps to the trailhead [1] after fully absorbing the beautiful views.

NATHAN GILMORE Originally from Ohio, Nathan Gilmore (1830–1898) settled on a ranch near Mud Springs, southeast of Placerville. Each summer he would pasture his angora goats around Fallen Leaf Lake. Angora goats, whose fleece is used to make mohair, weren't introduced to North America until the mid-1850s. Gilmore became a more notable figure after he discovered some mineral springs southwest of Fallen Leaf Lake. He built one of Tahoe's first resorts, which was originally known as Gilmore's Soda Springs (the name was later changed to Glen Alpine Springs after a poem by Sir Walter Scott to honor his recently deceased wife). Over the years, Gilmore developed the resort, constructing twenty-five buildings, including the social hall designed by notable architect Bernard Maybeck. Today, the Forest Service manages the old resort as a historic site.

To continue on to Angora Lakes, head southwest along the road, following a gently descending route across the ridge crest. At the base of a rise, the road shortly bends left to circumvent the hillside ahead. Abandoning the road for a direct route over the hill and picking up the road again on the far side is possible if you don't mind the stiff climb. Otherwise, follow the road on a gentle, arcing descent around the hill. On the far side, the road bends again and starts a moderately steep climb up to the first and smallest Angora Lake [4]. Thankfully, snowmobiles are banned beyond this point.

If the course of the road gets hard to follow beyond the first lake, simply follow a set of utility lines running up the hillside to the summer homes on the north and east shores of the middle lake. The terrain levels and provides easy transport over the last 100 yards to the shoreline of middle Angora Lake [5].

To reach upper Angora Lake [6], head for the low notch through which a stream connects the two larger lakes. The two upper and larger Angora Lakes nestle in basins at the base of steep cliffs forming the east face of 8,588-foot Angora Peak and the northeast face of Echo Peak. Many private cabins ring the shorelines of both lakes, so please be respectful of the private property. At the conclusion of your visit, retrace your steps back to the trailhead [1].

MILESTONES

1: Start at trailhead; 2: Left at junction; 3: Angora Lookout; 4: Lower Angora Lake; 5: Middle Angora Lake; 6: Upper Angora Lake; 1: Return to trailhead.

GO GREEN | Snowlands Network is a fine organization dedicated to protecting winter human-powered recreation across public lands. Consult their website at www.snowlands.org.

OPTIONS | Unless you're an accomplished mountaineer bound for Echo Peak, there's really no place for mere mortals to go to get out of the lake's basin.

WARM-UPS | Mexican cuisine should provide a sure-fire way to warm up after a day in the snow, and Verde Mexican Rotisserie in the Crossing Shopping Center at the Y in South Lake Tahoe should adequately fill the bill. Open daily from 8 AM to 8 PM (4 PM on Sundays), owners Domi and Katy Chavarria feature wholesome and healthy meals. Call 530-573-0700 for more information, or visit their website at www.verdemexicanrotisserie.com to see their menu.

44 | Fallen Leaf Lake

The gentle terrain around Fallen Leaf Lake, lacking any significant relief, is well suited for novice snowshoers, or for more advanced users searching for an easy romp into the backcountry. The area is quite popular on weekends of good weather, when numerous Nordic skiers kick and glide on some of the trails around the lake. In addition to human-powered recreationists, snowmobiles are permitted to use land south of State Route 89 between Fallen Leaf Road and the Desolation Wilderness boundary.

When planning your visit, you can create trips of varying lengths to suit your individual needs and schedule. The minimum distance from the SNO-PARK to Fallen Leaf Lake is about 1.5 miles, but much longer trips are quite possible. The lakeshore offers fine views across the water to the rugged east faces of Mount Tallac and Cathedral Peak.

LEVEL	Novice
LENGTH	3 miles, out and back to Fallen Leaf Lake
TIME	3 hours
ELEVATION	Negligible
DIFFICULTY	Easy
AVALANCHE RISK	Low
DOGS	OK
FACILITIES	Port-a-potty
MAP	USGS *Emerald Bay*
MANAGEMENT	Lake Tahoe Basin Management Unit at 530-543-2600, www.fs.usda.gov/ltbmu
HIGHLIGHTS	Lake, scenery
LOWLIGHT	Low elevation

TIP | Camp Richardson nearby offers the opportunity, for a fee, to follow marked trails across their property (see Warm-ups section).

TRAILHEAD | 38°55.938'N, 120°03.462'W From the Y in South Lake Tahoe, where Highways 50 and 89 meet, drive north on State Route 89 for 3.3 miles

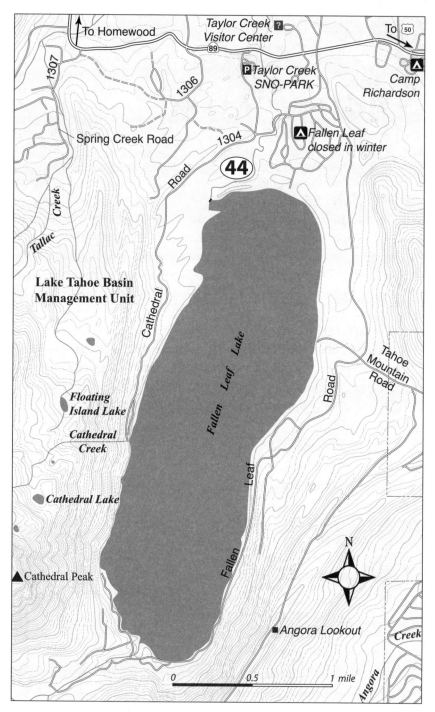

To Homewood

Taylor Creek
Visitor Center

89

1307

1306

Taylor Creek
SNO-PARK

To 50

Camp
Richardson

Spring Creek Road

1304

1304

Road

44

Fallen Leaf
closed in winter

Tallac Creek

Lake Tahoe Basin
Management Unit

Cathedral Road

Fallen Leaf Lake

Tahoe
Mountain
Road

Floating
Island Lake

Road

Cathedral
Creek

Leaf

Cathedral Lake

N

Cathedral Peak

Fallen

Angora Lookout

Creek

0   0.5   1 mile

Angora

44. Fallen Leaf Lake

to the access road to the Taylor Creek SNO-PARK, which is about a mile north of Camp Richardson. Follow the short road to the parking area.

ROUTE | A variety of possible routes radiate from the SNO-PARK around the north end of Fallen Leaf Lake. The most direct route will take you to the lake-shore in about three-quarters of a mile.

RACCOON (*Procyon lotor*) As omnivores, raccoons eat a diverse diet, in-cluding smaller animals, eggs, insects, and food from human sources. They store up layers of fat during autumn to prepare for the long snowy winters around Lake Tahoe, during which they can lose between 15 and 50 percent of their body weight. Their fur also grows thicker during winter. Although they do not hibernate, they may remain inside their warm dens for weeks, thanks to these fat stores. They prefer hollow trees for winter residences but will opportunistically use abandoned burrows of other animals, caves, or vacant buildings. Raccoons may be active in the winter, foraging for food during periods of warm weather.

GO GREEN | You can assist the Lake Tahoe Basin Management Unit of the Forest Service by volunteering your time through the Trees and Trails pro-gram, which offers a variety of opportunities for service. Visit www.fs.usda. gov/main/ltbmu/workingtogether/volunteering for further information.

OPTIONS | To spend the day exploring more of Fallen Leaf Lake, head along the north shore by following a route through the campground to Fallen Leaf Road and then go south past a large meadow on the right. Eventually, the road bends toward the shore of the lake, where there are fine views across the surface to Mount Tallac and Cathedral Peak. Although continuing south along the road is possible, most parties will head back to the trailhead where the road enters a neighborhood of summer homes on the southwest shore.

WARM-UPS | Camp Richardson is an all-year resort offering a number of possibil-ities for winter visitors. You can rent snowshoes or cross-country skis from the Mountain Sports Center and pay to use their marked system of groomed trails. Call 530-542-6584 to check conditions or for more information. A variety of lodging options is available for overnighters, with an assortment of packages.

The Beacon is a lakeshore restaurant at 1900 Jameson Beach Road offering daily dining options for lunch and dinner. Reservations (530-541-0630) are recommended on weekends. Visit the website at www.camprichardson.com for more information.

■ Additional Trips

HORSE MEADOWS: 38°47.480'N, 119°55.969'W Forest Road 051 departs from State Route 89, 1.7 miles northbound of Picketts Junction or 0.75 mile southbound of Luther Pass. Along with snowmobiles, you can travel this moderately graded road about 4.5 miles to Horse Meadows, from where you have a fine view of Freel Peak, the Tahoe Basin's highest summit.

HOPE VALLEY: 38°45.043'N, 119°56.392'W (SNO-PARK) Whether you park in the Hope Valley SNO-PARK or find a spot along the shoulder of either CA 89 or CA 88, the open plain of Hope Valley offers unlimited options for strolling across the open meadows.

CAPLES AND EMIGRANT LAKES: 38°42.199'N, 120°03.978'W From the vicinity of Caples Lake Dam, a pleasant route along the south shore of Caples Lake leads 2.5 miles to Emigrant Creek. From there, a more difficult journey follows Emigrant Creek to a dramatic cirque basin holding Emigrant Lake at 4.5 miles.

ECHO PEAK: 38°49.415'N, 120°02.031'W Another journey from the Echo Lakes SNO-PARK, a full-day trip follows the shoreline of Lower and Upper Echo Lakes to a stiff climb up the southwest slope of Echo Peak.

PART FOUR

WEST TAHOE

For purposes of this guide, West Tahoe covers an area roughly from Tahoe City south to Meeks Bay. Aside from the State Route 89 corridor, the west side is perhaps the most serene and peaceful shore of the lake, characterized by deep forests and trickling streams. A number of pleasant trips proceed alongside creeks lined with tall conifers, with many reaching pristine lakes or serene meadows.

Most of the routes in this chapter begin at an elevation near lake level, which generally limits the availability of a decent snowpack to the true months of snowy winters. Stanford Rock at 8,473 feet is the only destination even approaching a significantly high elevation. Consequently, snow conditions on the west shore may run the gamut from dry powder left over from a cold Pacific storm to wet, spring-like mush, or no snow at all. Thankfully, a moderate forest cover shades much of the area during the winter, which aids in hanging onto whatever snow may be present. Once the warmer temperatures and higher angle of the sun arrive in early spring, the snow line starts to creep up the hillside, eventually ending the snow season on this side of the lake.

Difficulty ratings for west side trips are easy to moderate, allowing plenty of opportunities for novice and intermediate snowshoers to explore the riches of Tahoe's backcountry. Aside from Stanford Rock, most of the trips travel across gentle terrain requiring minimal navigational skills.

Many of the trips follow well-established cross-country ski routes for at least part of the way. Westside trails have long been popular with the Nordic crowd, and sharing the path with these fellow winter travelers is a foregone conclusion. Remember to follow proper trail etiquette in commonly used areas. The initial segments of routes in Sugar Pine Point State Park and Blackwood Canyon are the two most likely areas where you're likely to encounter skiers. Unfortunately, snowmobiles are allowed in Blackwood Canyon.

■ Access

Access from State Route 89 to trailheads along the west shore is generally straightforward. Except for Meeks Creek and Page Meadows, the rest of the trails begin at either Sugar Pine Point State Park or the Blackwood Canyon SNO-PARK. Both areas provide plenty of parking and sanitation facilities, although both require a fee as well. Beware of attempting trips starting in other locations, as Placer County will issue citations for parking in residential areas and along county roads.

■ Communities

West shore communities with services for travelers between Tahoe City and Meeks Bay include Sunnyside, Tahoe Pines, and Homewood.

45 | Meeks Creek

Meeks Creek offers a fine haven when the weather is less than agreeable at the higher elevations. In addition, the essentially flat terrain is well suited for beginners who want to test out their "snow legs." The smooth surface of the valley extends upstream for about 1.5 miles before steeper topography leads into Desolation Wilderness.

LEVEL	Novice
LENGTH	3.6 miles, out and back
TIME	Half day
ELEVATION	Negligible
DIFFICULTY	Easy
AVALANCHE RISK	Low
DOGS	OK
FACILITIES	None
MAPS	USGS *Homewood*, *Meeks Bay*
MANAGEMENT	Lake Tahoe Basin Management Unit at 530-543-2600, www.fs.usda.gov/ltbmu
HIGHLIGHTS	Creek, meadow
LOWLIGHTS	Low elevation, parking

TIP | An early arrival may help the odds of securing a convenient parking space.

TRAILHEAD | 39°02.244'N, 120°07.560'W From the junction of Highway 28 in Tahoe City, head south on State Route 89 for 10.4 miles (or 15.3 miles north of the Y in South Lake Tahoe) and park along the highway as space allows.

ROUTE | [1] The route begins near an old wooden building and a Forest Service signboard. Pass over or around a gate and head southwest on the snow-covered course of FS 14N32. Continue up the broad valley, which offers fine views of the meadows lining Meeks Creek. Although the designated route follows the course of the road, the terrain is open enough to allow you to determine your own path up the valley. At the far end of the meadows, enter a substantial stand of trees. The road ends on top of a low rise [2], from where

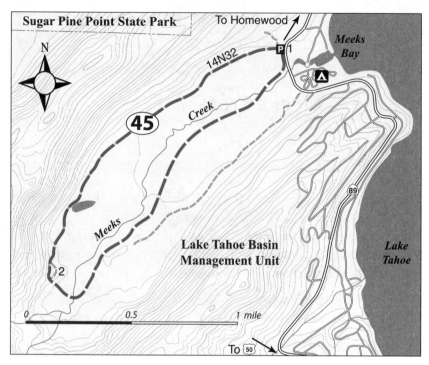

Sugar Pine Point State Park

To Homewood

Meeks Bay

N

14N32

P 1

Creek

45

Meeks

Lake Tahoe Basin
Management Unit

2

Lake Tahoe

89

0   0.5   1 mile

To 50

45. Meeks Creek

you have limited views farther up the canyon. The rise is a good spot for a break or lunch before heading back to your vehicle [1], as shortly beyond the rise, the terrain begins to steepen.

> **LONG-TAILED VOLE** (*Microtus longicaudus sierrae*) Voles are common residents of meadows and streamside environments, subsisting primarily on the lush grasses, sedges, and forbs found in those communities. They are prolific breeders.

MILESTONES

1: Start at trailhead; 2: Top of rise; 1: Return to trailhead.

GO GREEN | Snowlands Network is a fine organization dedicated to protecting winter human-powered recreation across public lands. Consult their website at www.snowlands.org.

OPTIONS | If you can find a safe way to cross Meeks Creek, you can alter your return by snowshoeing along the south side of the creek back toward the

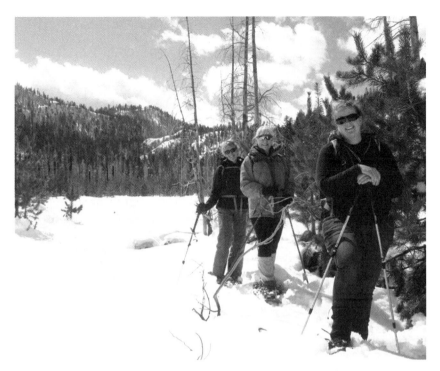
Snowshoers enjoying the scenery at Meeks Creek

highway. The highway bridge can be used to get back over the creek to return to your vehicle.

WARM-UPS | Obexer's General Store in Homewood at 5300 West Lake Boulevard has a deli that makes some of the best sandwiches at the lake. They also have breakfast burritos and bagel breakfast sandwiches until 11:00 AM. Visit their website at www.obexersgeneralstore.com.

Ed Z'berg Sugar Pine Point State Park

Snowshoers searching for the combination of pleasant scenery, gentle terrain, and marked trails will find this California state park an answer to their dreams. The park offers a fine network of designated routes that travel over essentially level terrain, two on serenely forested trails to the west of State Route 89 and two on the east side that offer lake views and a bit of California history.

TRAILHEAD | 39°02.985'N 120°06.892'W Head south from Tahoe City on State Route 89 for about 9 miles from the junction of Highway 28 to the vicinity of Ed Z'berg Sugar Pine Point State Park. Continue to the south entrance, turn left, and proceed shortly to the parking lot.

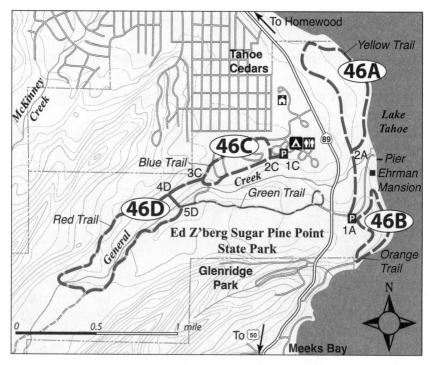

46A, B, C, D. Ed Z'berg Sugar Pine Point State Park

LEVEL Novice

LENGTH 2 miles, lollipop loop

TIME 2 hours

ELEVATION Negligible

DIFFICULTY Easy

AVALANCHE RISK Low

DOGS Not allowed except in parking area on leash

FACILITIES Campground, park office, restrooms, snowshoe tours

MAPS USGS *Meeks Bay, Homewood*; CSP *Ed Z'berg Sugar Pine Point State Park Cross-Country Ski Map* (available from park office or website, www.parks.ca.gov/pages/510/files /EdZSugarPinePtSkiTrailMapWinter2011.pdf)

MANAGEMENT California State Parks at 530-525-7982, www.parks.ca.gov

HIGHLIGHTS History, lake views

LOWLIGHTS Fee, low elevation

ROUTE | [1A] From the south parking area, head north on the Yellow Trail, cross General Creek, and then reach the loop junction [2A]. Turn right and follow the path to the shore of Lake Tahoe and continue north toward the park boundary, enjoying fine views of the lake and mountains along the way. Approaching the edge of park property, the trail arcs back around to the south and closes the loop section at the junction [2A]. From there, retrace your steps to the trailhead [1A].

MILESTONES

1A: Start at trailhead; 2A: Right at junction; 2A: Straight at junction; 1A: Return to trailhead.

LEVEL Novice

LENGTH 1.2 miles, loop

TIME 1 hour

ELEVATION Negligible

DIFFICULTY Easy

AVALANCHE RISK Low

DOGS Not allowed except in parking area on leash

FACILITIES Campground, park office, restrooms, snowshoe tours

MAPS USGS *Meeks Bay, Homewood*; CSP *Ed Z'berg Sugar Pine Point State Park Cross-Country Ski Map* (available from

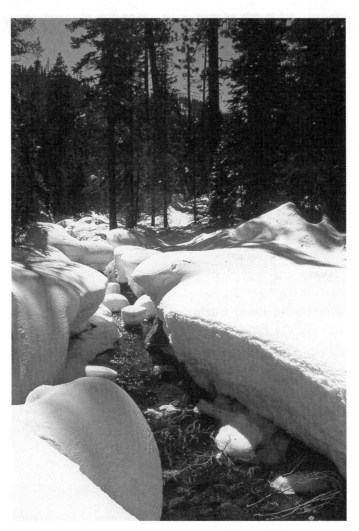

General Creek

park office or website, www.parks.ca.gov/pages/510/files
/EdZSugarPinePtSkiTrailMapWinter2011.pdf)

MANAGEMENT California State Parks at 530-525-7982, www.parks.ca.gov

HIGHLIGHTS History, lake views

LOWLIGHTS Fee, low elevation

ROUTE | [1A] From the parking area, follow the Orange Trail south to begin a counterclockwise loop through the forest toward the park boundary. Reach the shore of Lake Tahoe and bend around to the north. Pass by the South Boathouse and enjoy beautiful lake views on the way toward Pine Lodge (Ehrman Mansion). Just before the mansion grounds, the route bends sharply south again and soon closes the loop [1A].

LEVEL	Novice
LENGTH	2.1 miles, loop
TIME	2 hours
ELEVATION	Negligible
DIFFICULTY	Easy
AVALANCHE RISK	Low
DOGS	Not allowed except in parking area on leash
FACILITIES	Campground, park office, restrooms, snowshoe tours
MAPS	USGS *Meeks Bay, Homewood*; CSP *Ed Z'berg Sugar Pine Point State Park Cross-Country Ski Map* (available from park office or website, www.parks.ca.gov/pages/510/files /EdZSugarPinePtSkiTrailMapWinter2011.pdf)
MANAGEMENT	California State Parks at 530-525-7982, www.parks.ca.gov
HIGHLIGHT	Forest
LOWLIGHTS	Fee, low elevation

ROUTE | [1C] From the parking area, follow the Blue Trail through moderate forest cover on the way to the first junction [2C]. Maps have been placed at each major junction, which makes traveling through the park straightforward for all levels. Bear right at the junction and proceed on a counterclockwise circuit through the trees. Near the halfway point, you reach a junction [3C] between the Blue and Red Trails. Veer ahead on the left-hand trail and follow the loop back to the first junction [2C]. From there, retrace your steps shortly to the trailhead [1C].

MILESTONES

1C: Start at trailhead; 2C: Right at junction; 3C: Straight at junction; 2C: Straight at junction; 1C: Return to trailhead.

LEVEL	Intermediate
LENGTH	3.3 miles, lollipop loop
TIME	Half day
ELEVATION	Negligible
DIFFICULTY	Moderate
AVALANCHE RISK	Low
DOGS	Not allowed except in parking area on leash
FACILITIES	Campground, park office, restrooms, snowshoe tours
MAPS	USGS *Meeks Bay, Homewood*; CSP *Ed Z'berg Sugar Pine Point State Park Cross-Country Ski Map* (available from

park office or website, www.parks.ca.gov/pages/510/files /EdZSugarPinePtSkiTrailMapWinter2011.pdf)

MANAGEMENT California State Parks at 530-525-7982, www.parks.ca.gov

HIGHLIGHT Forest

LOWLIGHTS Fee, low elevation

ROUTE | [1C] From the parking area, follow the Blue Trail through moderate forest cover on the way to the first junction [2C]. Maps have been placed at each major junction, which makes traveling through the park straightforward for all levels. Bear right at the junction and proceed on a counterclockwise circuit through the trees. Near the halfway point of the Blue Trail, you reach a junction [3C] with the Red Trail. Veer right from the junction and follow the Red Trail upstream along the north bank of General Creek, passing a small meadow on the way to the loop junction [4D].

Go straight (right) and head southwest above the north bank of General Creek. Reach a bridge over the creek at the far end of the loop. Here the forest lightens, allowing limited views of the surrounding terrain near Olympic Meadows, site of the 1960 Olympic Biathlon Range. Now heading northeast along the south bank, you eventually reach a junction [5D] with the Green Trail on your right. Turn left here, cross another bridge over General Creek, and proceed to the next junction [4D]. From there, turn right and simply retrace your steps along the Red and Blue Trails to the parking area [1C].

MILESTONES

1C: Start at trailhead; 2C: Right at junction; 3C: Right at junction; 4D: Straight at loop junction; 5D: Left at Green Trail junction; 4D: Right at loop junction; 1C: Return to trailhead.

GO GREEN | Volunteers are essential in the California State Park system. Opportunities include docents, visitor center volunteers, public safety, operations,

HELLMAN-EHRMAN MANSION The centerpiece of the park is assuredly the stately mansion near the shore of Lake Tahoe. I. W. Hellman, a San Francisco businessman, began accumulating property in the area beginning in 1897. By 1913, he had acquired almost 2,000 acres. By 1903, artisans had completed Pine Lodge, his summer home. His daughter, Florence Hellman Ehrman, inherited the mansion, along with her husband, Sydney. They spent numerous summers there. The mansion and 1,975 acres of land became property of California State Parks in 1965. During the summer, daily tours of the mansion are offered to the general public.

maintenance, administration, and natural and cultural resource protection. For more information, visit the state park website at www.parks.ca.gov/?page_ id=886, call 916-653-9069, or email: volunteer.inparksprogram@parks.ca.gov.

OPTIONS | More adventurous souls can opt for a much longer journey upstream along General Creek and then south out of the canyon on a mile-plus-long, 1,000-foot climb to Lost and Duck Lakes (see Map 46E Lost Lake and Duck Lake). From the end of the Red Trail loop, continue upstream along General Creek for about a mile to the vicinity of a tributary that drains the lakes to the south. Climb up this drainage, steeply at times, to a bench holding the frozen lakes.

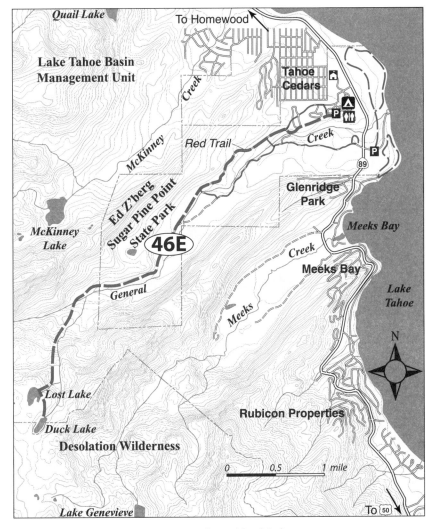

46E. Lost Lake and Duck Lake

WARM-UPS | Winter campers can set up a base camp within a plowed area inside Ed Z'berg Sugar Pine Point State Park near the north entrance. Fees are $25 per night and although the showers are closed for the season, the park has a central-heated restroom with potable water. Campers can use the fire pits, picnic tables, and food lockers, but campers are responsible for shoveling them out.

Jake's on the Lake has been serving west Lake Tahoe since 1978 at 780 N. Lake Boulevard in Tahoe City. Dishes with fresh seafood, quality meats, and seasonal produce are served for lunch on winter weekends from 11:30 AM and dinner nightly starting at 5:00 PM. Recreationists will find the casual atmosphere a fine complement to their fresh cuisine and stunning lake view. To view menus or for more information, visit their website at www.jakestahoe .com, or phone 530-583-0188 for reservations.

McKinney, Lily, and Miller Lakes and Miller Meadows

Most of this route follows the alignment of a section of the McKinney-Rubicon OHV Road past three good-size lakes to expansive Miller Meadows. Due to wintertime parking restrictions where the road begins in the summer, human-powered winter enthusiasts are forced to begin the trip inside Ed Z'berg Sugar Pine Point State Park and then climb over the ridge forming the north side of General Creek canyon to access the snow-covered road. Crossing the ridge is the most difficult part of the journey physically and will also necessitate a bit of route finding. Once in the McKinney Creek drainage, the route follows a gentle grade upstream to the lakes and meadows.

LEVEL	Advanced
LENGTH	7 miles to McKinney Lake, out and back; 12 miles to Miller Meadows, out and back
TIME	Full day
ELEVATION	+1,050'–775'
DIFFICULTY	Moderate to strenuous
AVALANCHE RISK	Moderate
DOGS	Not allowed except in parking area on leash
FACILITIES	Campground, park office, restrooms, snowshoe tours
MAPS	USGS *Meeks Bay, Homewood*; CSP *Ed Z'berg Sugar Pine Point State Park Cross-Country Ski Map* (available from park office or website, www.parks.ca.gov/pages/510/files /EdZSugarPinePtSkiTrailMapWinter2011.pdf)
MANAGEMENT	California State Parks at 530-525-7982, www.parks.ca.gov; Lake Tahoe Basin Management Unit at 530-543-2600, www.fs.usda.gov/ltbmu
HIGHLIGHTS	Forest, meadows, lakes
LOWLIGHTS	Fee, low elevation

TIP | Once on the McKinney-Rubicon OHV Road, keep alert for snowmobiles.

TRAILHEAD | 39°03.431'N, 120°07.354'W Head south from Tahoe City on State Route 89 for about 9 miles from the junction of Highway 28 to the vicinity of Ed Z'berg Sugar Pine Point State Park. Turn right from the highway at the north entrance and proceed shortly to the parking area.

ROUTE | [1] From the parking area, follow the Blue Trail through moderate forest cover on the way to the first junction [2]. Maps have been placed at each major junction, which makes traveling through the park straightforward for all levels. Bear right at the junction and proceed on a counterclockwise circuit through the trees. Near the halfway point of the Blue Trail, you reach a junction [3] with the Red Trail.

Leave the designated trail near the junction and head generally west on a moderate ascent toward the top of a ridge. Ideally, you want to intersect a road just below Peak 6814 at about one and a quarter mile from the parking area. Follow this road briefly to the ridge crest separating the drainages of General and McKinney Creeks. Remain on the road on a descent toward McKinney Creek. Reach the McKinney-Rubicon OHV Road [4] in the bottom of the canyon near the 2-mile mark.

Turn upstream and follow the road through gentle, forested terrain, crossing McKinney Creek after about a mile and then a tributary draining Buck Lake a half mile farther. A short way past the second stream, the road starts to curve around a hillside below Peak 7534 and then passes above McKinney Lake, 3.5 miles from the trailhead. The lake is relatively large and is surrounded by dense forest at the base of the ridge. To reach the lakeshore, you'll have to descend a steep hillside to access the north shore [5].

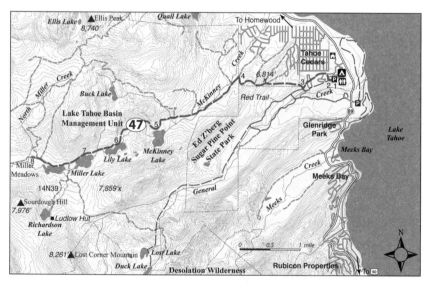

47. McKinney, Lily, and Miller Lakes and Miller Meadows

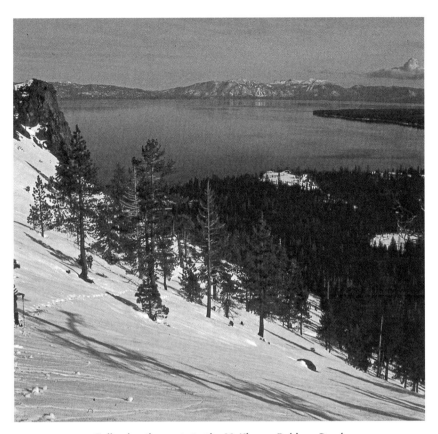

Following the route to the McKinney-Rubicon Road

LUDLOW HUT Managed by the Sierra Club, the Ludlow Hut has a main living area with wood-burning stove, tables, and a kitchen. Overnighters can bunk in the upstairs loft, which can accommodate up to fifteen guests. A separate two-story outhouse is about 100 feet to the southeast. Volunteers built the hut in 1955 as a memorial to William B. Ludlow (1930–1953), a Berkeley native, Sierra Club member, and lover of the outdoors. He was killed in a tragic accident while serving in the Corps of Engineers during the Korean War. For information about reserving the hut, contact the Sierra Club at Clair Tappaan Lodge (http://clairtappaanlodge.com). Hut reservations are accepted by phone (530-426-3632 from 9:00 AM to 5:00 PM) or by email (reservations@clairtappaanlodge.com). The lodge's mailing address is PO Box 36, Norden, CA 95724). For more information about the hut, visit http://clairtappaanlodge.com/ludlow-hut.

Away from McKinney Lake, a gentle, mile-long climb leads to Lily Lake [6], long and narrow, and like McKinney perched below a ridge and surrounded by trees.

From Lily Lake, an easy half-mile stroll brings you to the next body of water, Miller Lake [7], at 5 miles from the trailhead. Tree-lined as well, Miller is a large lake with a pair of hills above the far shore.

From the east edge of Miller Lake, another half mile of easy travel brings you to the beginning of Miller Meadows [8], 5.5 miles from the parking area, which are composed of two expansive clearings separated by a grove of trees. The area offers wide-ranging opportunities for further exploration of the meadows and surrounding terrain. Sourdough Hill stands guard over the meadows and provides a reliable landmark for those desiring to expand their journey farther to Richardson Lake (see Options section). When the time comes, retrace your steps to the trailhead [1].

MILESTONES

1: Start at trailhead; 2: Right at junction; 3: Leave marked trail; 4: Left at McKinney-Rubicon OHV Road; 5: McKinney Lake; 6: Lily Lake; 7: Miller Lake; 8: Miller Meadows; 1: Return to trailhead.

GO GREEN | Keep Tahoe Blue has been active at Lake Tahoe for sixty years, advocating, educating, and collaborating to protect the quality of the lake's environment. Consult their website at www.keeptahoeblue.org.

OPTIONS | Although doing so would make a long day even longer, extending the trip south to Richardson Lake is a viable option. From the west end of Miller Lake, either follow the course of FS 14N39 or the drainage of Richardson Lake's outlet generally south for a mile of moderate climbing through mixed forest. Determining the actual location of the fair-sized lake should be reasonably straightforward, resting in a bowl between Sourdough Hill and Lost Corner Mountain. Overnighters can make reservations to stay at the Sierra Club's Ludlow Hut above the east shore.

WARM-UPS | Obexer's General Store In Homewood at 5300 West Lake Boulevard has a deli that makes some of the best sandwiches at the lake. They also have breakfast burritos and bagel breakfast sandwiches until 11:00 AM. Visit their website at www.obexersgeneralstore.com.

TRIP
48 | Buck Lake

A secluded lake off the beaten path is the goal of this trip. You may see other recreationists along the section of this route that follows the McKinney-Rubicon OHV Road, but once you leave the road, most, if not all, will disappear. The lake is quite scenic, a worthy destination set quietly in a long, flat basin nearly enclosed by precipitous cliffs.

LEVEL	Advanced
LENGTH	10 miles, out and back
TIME	Three-quarter day
ELEVATION	+1,425'–275'
DIFFICULTY	Moderate
AVALANCHE RISK	Moderate
DOGS	Not allowed except in parking area on leash
FACILITIES	Campground, park office, restrooms, snowshoe tours
MAPS	USGS *Meeks Bay*, *Homewood*; CSP *Ed Z'berg Sugar Pine Point State Park Cross-Country Ski Map* (available from park office or website, www.parks.ca.gov/pages/510/files /EdZSugarPinePtSkiTrailMapWinter2011.pdf)
MANAGEMENT	California State Parks at 530-525-7982, www.parks.ca.gov; Lake Tahoe Basin Management Unit at 530-543-2600, www.fs.usda.gov/ltbmu
HIGHLIGHTS	Forest, lake
LOWLIGHTS	Fee, low elevation

TIP | Once on the McKinney-Rubicon OHV Road, keep alert for snowmobiles.

TRAILHEAD | 39°03.431'N, 120°07.354'W Head south from Tahoe City on State Route 89 for about 9 miles from the junction of Highway 28 to the vicinity of Ed Z'berg Sugar Pine Point State Park. Turn right from the highway at the north entrance and proceed shortly to the parking area.

ROUTE | [1] From the parking area, follow the Blue Trail through moderate forest cover on the way to the first junction [2]. Maps have been placed at each major junction, which makes traveling through the park straightforward for all levels. Bear left at the junction and proceed on a counterclockwise circuit through the trees. Near the halfway point of the Blue Trail, you reach a junction [3] with the Red Trail.

Leave the marked trail near the junction and head generally west on a moderate ascent toward the top of a ridge. Ideally, you want to intersect a road just below Peak 6814 at about one and a quarter mile from the parking area. Follow this road briefly to the ridge crest separating the drainages of General and McKinney Creeks. Remain on the road on a descent toward McKinney Creek. Reach the McKinney-Rubicon OHV Road [4] in the bottom of the canyon near the 2-mile mark.

Turn upstream and follow the road through gentle, forested terrain, crossing McKinney Creek after about a mile and then a tributary [5] draining Buck Lake a half mile farther.

Leave the McKinney-Rubicon Road at the creek and turn northwest up the drainage on a moderately steep climb. Bear left where the slope is more moderate to gain a four-wheel-drive road generally paralleling the stream. Continue climbing moderately up the road, passing in and out of light forest. A final stretch of climbing brings you well above the long valley holding Bucks Lake. A moderately steep descent from the road leads to the lakeshore [6].

Buck Lake occupies a small part of a long and narrow basin rimmed by steep cliffs. With a coat of winter white, the lake is almost indiscernible from the smooth valley floor. The surroundings create a very pleasant place to rest and enjoy the scenery before heading back to the trailhead [1].

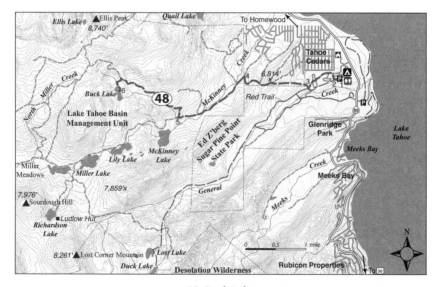

48. Buck Lake

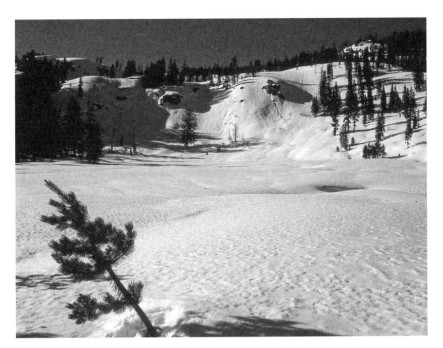

Buck Lake

MILESTONES

1: Start at trailhead; 2: Right at junction; 3: Leave marked trail; 4: Left at McKinney-Rubicon OHV Road; 5: Right at outlet from Buck Lake; 6: Buck Lake; 1: Return to trailhead.

GO GREEN | Snowlands Network is a fine organization dedicated to protecting winter human-powered recreation across public lands. Consult their website at www.snowlands.org.

OPTIONS | The trip to Buck Lake and back should be enough for most recreationists for one day.

WARM-UPS | Obexer's General Store In Homewood at 5300 West Lake Boulevard has a deli that makes some of the best sandwiches at the lake. They also have breakfast burritos and bagel breakfast sandwiches until 11:00 AM. Visit their website at www.obexersgeneralstore.com.

AMERICAN (PINE) MARTEN (*Martes americana*) A member of the weasel family, this secretive mammal prefers a habitat of mature, dense forest with a thick canopy. They are active during the winter and do not hibernate. Their diet typically consists of rodents.

TRIP

49 Stanford Rock

On weekends of ample snow and good weather, outdoor enthusiasts, including snowmobilers, heavily use the Blackwood Canyon SNO-PARK for setting off on their adventures. For snowshoers who don't mind the road less traveled, they can leave the masses behind right from the beginning of this trip to Stanford Rock. With the exception of the steep ascent at the beginning necessary to gain the ridge that forms the north side of Blackwood Canyon, the majority of the route climbs manageably at a moderate grade. Occasional views through breaks in the forest along the way are outdone by the sweeping view of Lake Tahoe above the sheer north face of Stanford Rock, along with the peaks and ridges surrounding Blackwood Canyon.

LEVEL	Advanced
LENGTH	7 miles, out and back
TIME	Three-quarter day
ELEVATION	+2,200'–0'
DIFFICULTY	Moderate
AVALANCHE RISK	Moderate
DOGS	OK
FACILITIES	Port-a-potty
MAP	USGS *Homewood*
MANAGEMENT	Lake Tahoe Basin Management Unit at 530-543-2600, www.fs.usda.gov/ltbmu
HIGHLIGHTS	Forest, summit, views
LOWLIGHTS	Low elevation, snowmobiles

TIP | The open slopes below Peak 7277, beginning one-third mile from the SNO-PARK, are covered with boulders and brush. This southern exposure is prone to soft conditions during sunny and warm periods, requiring you to watch your step, particularly in the afternoon. When avalanche conditions are a concern, ascend to the ridge crest on the forested slopes about a half mile farther up the canyon.

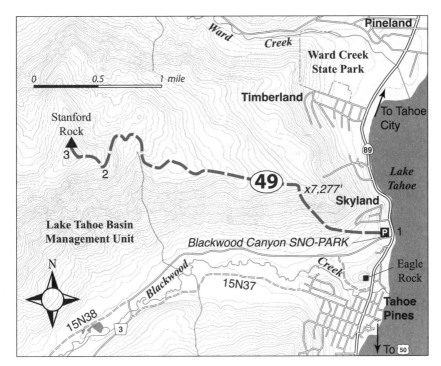

49. Stanford Rock

TRAILHEAD | 39°06.828'N, 120°09.509'W Travel south on State Route 89 for 4 miles from the junction of Highway 28 in Tahoe City to the well-marked entrance to the Blackwood Canyon SNO-PARK and Kaspian Recreation Area. Turn west and follow signs the short distance to the parking lot.

ROUTE | [1] Avoiding the well-traveled road, head directly west from the SNO-PARK into dense forest cover, staying away from the homes in the neighborhood to the north. After one-third mile of gentle snowshoeing, you reach a large clearing below the slopes of Peak 7277. A stiff climb leads away from the clearing on an arcing ascent to the northwest across a forested hillside toward the crest of the ridge above. Good views behind you of Lake Tahoe occur at times on this moderately steep climb, with Eagle Rock providing a fine accent to the emerald waters. About a mile from the trailhead, you encounter gentler terrain at the ridge crest amid a light mixed forest.

Heading generally west, follow the gently ascending ridgeline with occasional short moderate pitches for half a mile to a knob, from where there are excellent views of Blackwood Canyon (Lake Tahoe is blocked by trees). Continue along the ridge for another one-quarter mile to a snow-covered road, which is the route of a lightly used cross-country ski route from Ward Canyon to the north and a major mountain biking route in the summer. You

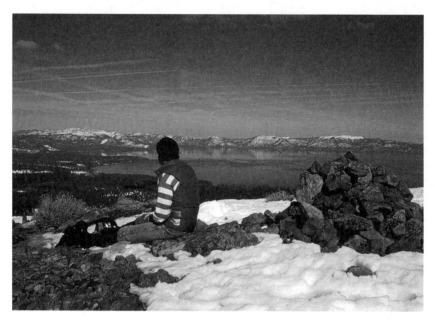

View from the top of Stanford Rock

can follow the road, which is easy to discern through the cut in the forest, or take a more direct route along the ridge.

The road option winds along the ridge for another one and a quarter miles through moderate forest cover to a viewpoint [2] offering exceptional vistas of Tahoe and a slice of Blackwood Canyon. From there, the road turns northwest and climbs the last one-quarter mile to the top of Stanford Rock [3].

Standing on the wind-blown rocks above the sheer north face of Stanford Rock, you gaze at the full majesty of Lake Tahoe. To the north is the backside of Alpine Meadows, flanked by Scott and Ward Peaks. The dramatic-looking form of Twin Peaks guards the upper reaches of Blackwood Canyon at the west end of the ridge. After thoroughly enjoying the view, retrace your steps back to the trailhead [1].

BALD EAGLE (*Haliaeetus leucocephalus*) Although far from a common sight in the skies above Lake Tahoe, bald eagles are occasionally seen during the winter months. The characteristic white or "bald" head does not appear until the birds are about five years old. Despite a wingspan of up to seven feet that makes them appear to be quite large birds, bald eagles only weigh between 10 and 14 pounds. When not nesting, they tend to be quite communal, with large groups roosting in tall trees.

1: Start at trailhead; 2: Viewpoint; 3: Stanford Rock; 1: Return to trailhead.

GO GREEN | You can assist the Lake Tahoe Basin Management Unit of the Forest Service by volunteering your time through the Trees and Trails program, which offers a variety of opportunities for service. Visit www.fs.usda.gov /main/ltbmu/workingtogether/volunteering for further information.

OPTIONS | Strong snowshoers have the option of adding Twin Peaks to the journey. Follow the ridge southwest from Stanford Rock to the base of the east peak. The final slope to the summit is steep and may be difficult, depending on snow conditions.

WARM-UPS | Sunnyside Restaurant and Lodge has been serving Tahoe residents and guests for many years. Light fare can be ordered in the Mountain Grill during lunch and dinner hours, while the Lakeside Dining Room offers more upscale cuisine for dinner only. The twenty-three guestrooms provide fine accommodations for those who want to enjoy an overnight stay. Check out their website at www.sunnysideresort.com.

TRIP

50 | Page Meadows

Page Meadows is a handful of clearings strung together to the north of Ward Creek. The nearly level terrain and short distance make this an easy trip for snowshoers of all levels. A minimal amount of route finding is necessary in order to reach the first meadow, but the route is so popular with locals that finding a beaten path is a pretty sure bet, unless you're the first one here after a storm. Once the first meadow is located, the rest of the clearings are easy to find. The open meadows provide pleasant scenery, well complemented by numerous aspen stands along the fringes.

LEVEL	Novice
LENGTH	3 miles, out and back (shorter trips possible)
TIME	3 hours
ELEVATION	Negligible
DIFFICULTY	Easy
AVALANCHE RISK	Low
DOGS	OK
FACILITIES	None
MAP	USGS *Tahoe City*
MANAGEMENT	Lake Tahoe Basin Management Unit at 530-543-2600, www.fs.usda.gov/ltbmu
HIGHLIGHTS	Forest, meadows
LOWLIGHT	Low elevation

TIP | Although the route to Page Meadows and back is fairly straightforward, there are a couple of ways to get lost. Navigation may be difficult if you happen to arrive right after a storm and there are no tracks to follow. Conversely, as the area is quite popular, a lot of tracks can also make route finding difficult if you're not paying attention.

TRAILHEAD | 39°08.776'N, 120°10.394'W In the lakeshore community of Sunnyside, about 2 miles south of the junction of Highway 28 in Tahoe City, leave State Route 89 and turn southwest onto Pine Avenue. After 0.2 mile, turn right on Tahoe Park Heights and drive 0.7 mile to the top of a hill and

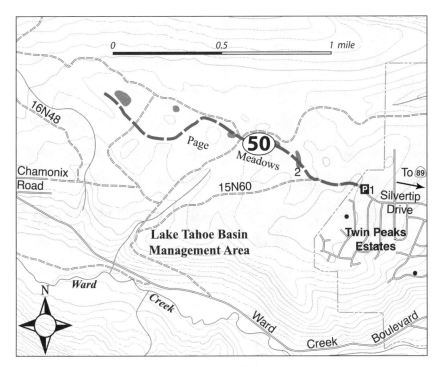

50. Page Meadows

a four-way intersection. Take the middle road, Big Pine Drive, and proceed one-quarter mile to a left-hand turn onto Silver Tip Drive. Follow Silver Tip to the end of the road and the signed parking area.

ROUTE | [1] Head west from the parking area on the unplowed continuation of the road through predominantly fir forest with lesser amounts of lodgepole pine and Jeffrey pine. After a gentle 0.1-mile climb, you reach a crest and then begin to descend for another 0.2 mile. Leave the road here and veer northwest, reaching the first meadow [2] in about 100 yards. From the north end of the first meadow, the route generally goes west-northwest through the other meadows. From whatever turnaround point you choose, retrace your steps back to the trailhead [1].

RED-TAILED HAWK (*Buteo jamaicenses*) Unlike bald eagles and ospreys, red-tailed hawks are fairly common sights in the Tahoe skies. Even when they're not visible, you may hear their characteristic high-pitched, descending screech echoing through the forest. In flight, its rust-colored tail easily identifies this large raptor.

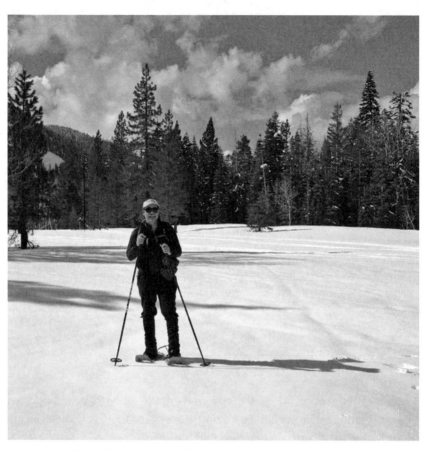

The author in Page Meadows. Photo by Amen Photography.

MILESTONES

1: Start at trailhead; **2:** First meadow; **1:** Return to trailhead.

GO GREEN | The Truckee River Watershed Council is a nonprofit organization dedicated to restoration of the watershed through research, management, funding, and education. To learn more about their work, consult their website at www.truckeeriverwc.org.

OPTIONS | Those looking for more of an outing than the gentle romp through Page Meadows could choose to head for Scott Peak to the west-northwest.

WARM-UPS | The Fire Sign Café in Tahoe City has been a local hot spot for breakfast and lunch since 1978. The restaurant is usually very busy on weekends, but the freshly prepared dishes are worth the wait. Not only will you find standard breakfast fare like bacon and eggs, but also more exotic dishes like the Cape Cod Benedict and the smoked salmon omelette. Both breakfast and lunch are served all day from 7:00 AM to 3:00 PM. The café occupies an old home at 1785 W. Lake Boulevard, about 2 miles south of the center of town. Visit their website at www.firesigncafe.com or phone 530-583-0871 for more information.

Additional Trips

BLACKWOOD CANYON: 39°06.828'N, 120°09.509'W Open to snowmobiles, the Barker Pass Road follows a gentle grade through the lower part of Blackwood Canyon, before climbing more steeply toward Barker Pass. Snowshoers can easily tailor the length and difficulty of a trip along the road to suit their needs.

Index

About the Author

Mike White grew up in Portland, Oregon, from where he began adventuring in the Cascade Range. He obtained a BA from Seattle Pacific University, where he met and married his wife, Robin. The couple lived in Seattle for two years before relocating to Reno. For the next fifteen years, Mike worked for a consulting engineering firm, journeying to the Sierra Nevada and other western ranges as time permitted. Upon leaving the engineering firm, Mike started writing full-time. A nationally award-winning author, Mike has contributed to numerous outdoor guides and has written many magazine and newspaper articles. He has published *50 Classic Hikes in Nevada*, *Best Backpacking Trips in California and Nevada* and *Best Backpacking Trips in Utah, Arizona and New Mexico* for the University of Nevada Press. A former community college instructor, Mike is also a featured speaker for outdoors and conservation organizations.